T0234542

OTHER FAST FACTS BOOKS

Fast Facts on **ADOLESCENT HEALTH FOR NURSING AND HEALTH PROFESSIONALS**: A Care Guide *(Herrman)*

Fast Facts for the **ANTEPARTUM AND POSTPARTUM NURSE**: A Nursing Orientation and Care Guide *(Davidson)*

Fast Facts Workbook for **CARDIAC DYSRHYTHMIAS AND 12-LEAD EKGs** *(Desmarais)*

Fast Facts for the **CARDIAC SURGERY NURSE**: Caring for Cardiac Surgery Patients, Third Edition *(Hodge)*

Fast Facts for **CAREER SUCCESS IN NURSING**: Making the Most of Mentoring *(Vance)*

Fast Facts for the **CATH LAB NURSE** *(McCulloch)*

Fast Facts for the **CLASSROOM NURSING INSTRUCTOR**: Classroom Teaching *(Yoder-Wise, Kowalski)*

Fast Facts for the **CLINICAL NURSE LEADER** *(Wilcox, Deerhake)*

Fast Facts for the **CLINICAL NURSE MANAGER**: Managing a Changing Workplace, Second Edition *(Fry)*

Fast Facts for the **CLINICAL NURSING INSTRUCTOR**: Clinical Teaching, Third Edition *(Kan, Stabler-Haas)*

Fast Facts on **COMBATING NURSE BULLYING, INCIVILITY, AND WORKPLACE VIOLENCE**: What Nurses Need to Know *(Ciocco)*

Fast Facts for the **CRITICAL CARE NURSE**, Second Edition *(Hewett)*

Fast Facts About **CURRICULUM DEVELOPMENT IN NURSING**: How to Develop and Evaluate Educational Programs, Second Edition *(McCoy, Anema)*

Fast Facts for **DEMENTIA CARE**: What Nurses Need to Know, Second Edition *(Miller)*

Fast Facts for **DEVELOPING A NURSING ACADEMIC PORTFOLIO**: What You Really Need to Know *(Wittmann-Price)*

Fast Facts for **DNP ROLE DEVELOPMENT**: A Career Navigation Guide *(Menonna-Quinn, Tortorella Genova)*

Fast Facts About **EKGs FOR NURSES**: The Rules of Identifying EKGs *(Landrum)*

Fast Facts for the **ER NURSE**: Emergency Department Orientation, Third Edition *(Buettner)*

Fast Facts for **EVIDENCE-BASED PRACTICE IN NURSING**: Third Edition *(Godshall)*

Fast Facts for the **FAITH COMMUNITY NURSE**: Implementing FCN/Parish Nursing *(Hickman)*

Fast Facts About **FORENSIC NURSING**: What You Need to Know *(Scannell)*

Fast Facts for the **GERONTOLOGY NURSE**: A Nursing Care Guide *(Eliopoulos)*

Fast Facts About **GI AND LIVER DISEASES FOR NURSES**: What APRNs Need to Know *(Chaney)*

Fast Facts About the **GYNECOLOGICAL EXAM**: A Professional Guide for NPs, PAs, and Midwives, Second Edition *(Secor, Fantasia)*

Fast Facts in **HEALTH INFORMATICS FOR NURSES** *(Hardy)*

Fast Facts for **HEALTH PROMOTION IN NURSING**: Promoting Wellness *(Miller)*

Fast Facts for Nurses About **HOME INFUSION THERAPY**: The Expert's Best Practice Guide *(Gorski)*

Fast Facts for the **HOSPICE NURSE**: A Concise Guide to End-of-Life Care, Second Edition *(Wright)*

Fast Facts for the **L&D NURSE**: Labor & Delivery Orientation, Second Edition *(Groll)*

Fast Facts for the **LONG-TERM CARE NURSE**: What Nursing Home and Assisted Living Nurses Need to Know *(Eliopoulos)*

Fast Facts to **LOVING YOUR RESEARCH PROJECT**: A Stress-Free Guide for Novice Researchers in Nursing and Healthcare *(Marshall)*

Fast Facts for **MAKING THE MOST OF YOUR CAREER IN NURSING** *(Redulla)*

Fast Facts for **MANAGING PATIENTS WITH A PSYCHIATRIC DISORDER**: What RNs, NPs, and New Psych Nurses Need to Know *(Marshall)*

Fast Facts About **MEDICAL CANNABIS AND OPIOIDS**: Minimizing Opioid Use Through Cannabis *(Smith, Smith)*

Fast Facts for the **MEDICAL OFFICE NURSE**: What You Really Need to Know *(Richmeier)*

Fast Facts for the **MEDICAL–SURGICAL NURSE**: Clinical Orientation *(Ciocco)*

Fast Facts for the **NEONATAL NURSE**: A Nursing Orientation and Care Guide *(Davidson)*

Fast Facts About **NEUROCRITICAL CARE**: A Quick Reference for the Advanced Practice Provider *(McLaughlin)*

Fast Facts for the **NEW NURSE PRACTITIONER**: What You Really Need to Know, Second Edition *(Aktan)*

Fast Facts for **NURSE PRACTITIONERS:** Practice Essentials for Clinical Subspecialties (*Aktan*)

Fast Facts for the **NURSE PRECEPTOR**: Keys to Providing a Successful Preceptorship *(Ciocco)*

Fast Facts for the **NURSE PSYCHOTHERAPIST**: The Process of Becoming *(Jones, Tusaie)*

Fast Facts About **NURSING AND THE LAW**: Law for Nurses *(Grant, Ballard)*

Fast Facts About the **NURSING PROFESSION**: Historical Perspectives *(Hunt)*

Fast Facts for the **OPERATING ROOM NURSE**: An Orientation and Care Guide, Second Edition *(Criscitelli)*

Fast Facts for the **PEDIATRIC NURSE**: An Orientation Guide *(Rupert, Young)*

Fast Facts Handbook for **PEDIATRIC PRIMARY CARE:** A Guide for Nurse Practitioners and Physician Assistants (*Ruggiero, Ruggiero*)

Fast Facts About **PRESSURE ULCER CARE FOR NURSES**: How to Prevent, Detect, and Resolve Them *(Dziedzic)*

Fast Facts About **PTSD**: A Guide for Nurses and Other Health Care Professionals *(Adams)*

Fast Facts for the **RADIOLOGY NURSE**: An Orientation and Nursing Care Guide, Second Edition *(Grossman)*

Fast Facts About **RELIGION FOR NURSES**: Implications for Patient Care *(Taylor)*

Fast Facts for the **SCHOOL NURSE**: What You Need to Know, Third Edition *(Loschiavo)*

Fast Facts About **SEXUALLY TRANSMITTED INFECTIONS**: A Nurse's Guide to Expert Patient Care *(Scannell)*

Fast Facts for **STROKE CARE NURSING**: An Expert Care Guide, Second Edition *(Morrison)*

Fast Facts for the **STUDENT NURSE**: Nursing Student Success *(Stabler-Haas)*

Fast Facts About **SUBSTANCE USE DISORDERS**: What Every Nurse, APRN, and PA Needs to Know *(Marshall, Spencer)*

Fast Facts for the **TRAVEL NURSE**: Travel Nursing *(Landrum)*

Fast Facts for the **TRIAGE NURSE**: An Orientation and Care Guide, Second Edition *(Visser, Montejano)*

Fast Facts for the **WOUND CARE NURSE**: Practical Wound Management *(Kifer)*

Fast Facts for **WRITING THE DNP PROJECT**: Effective Structure, Content, and Presentation *(Christenbery)*

Forthcoming FAST FACTS Books

Fast Facts for the **ADULT-GERONTOLOGY ACUTE CARE NURSE PRACTITIONER** *(Carpenter)*

Fast Facts About **COMPETENCY-BASED EDUCATION IN NURSING**: How to Teach Competency Mastery *(Wittmann-Price, Gittings)*

Fast Facts for **CREATING A SUCCESSFUL TELEHEALTH SERVICE**: A How-to Guide for Nurse Practitioners *(Heidesch)*

Fast Facts About **DIVERSITY, EQUITY, AND INCLUSION** *(Davis)*

Fast Facts for the **ER NURSE**: Guide to a Successful Emergency Department Orientation, Fourth Edition *(Buettner)*

Fast Facts for the **L&D NURSE**: Labor & Delivery Orientation, Third Edition *(Groll)*

Fast Facts About **LGBTQ CARE FOR NURSES** *(Traister)*

Fast Facts for the **NEONATAL NURSE**: Care Essentials for Normal and High-Risk Neonates, Second Edition *(Davidson)*

Fast Facts for the **NURSE PRECEPTOR**: Keys to Providing a Successful Preceptorship, Second Edition *(Ciocco)*

Fast Facts for **PATIENT SAFETY IN NURSING** *(Hunt)*

Visit www.springerpub.com to order.

FAST FACTS for
THE RADIOLOGY NURSE

Valerie Aarne Grossman, MALS, BSN, NE-BC, is an RN who has been serving in the healthcare industry for more than four decades. She has diverse work experience, including serving in small hospitals to large university medical centers and working in areas of healthcare such as emergency, critical care, telephone triage, pediatrics, radiology, and nursing leadership. She volunteers her time to support professional organizations such as the Emergency Nurses Association and the Association for Radiologic & Imaging Nursing. She has a long history of board service, supporting patient advocacy, Research Subjects Review Board (RSRB), nursing certification, and nursing journals, and is the chairperson for the New York State Board for Nursing from 2019 to 2021. She is the author of numerous peer-reviewed books, chapters, and articles and serves as a manuscript reviewer for a number of international publishers. Her passion for direct patient caregivers drives her involvement in projects that improve the tools, evidence-based information, and the regulations that affect those caring for patients. She believes that healthcare providers (especially nurses) are "scientists who touch patients" as well as "scientists who *are touched* by patients" and works to provide the intellectual information that feeds their professional curiosity.

FAST FACTS for
THE RADIOLOGY NURSE

An Orientation and Nursing Care Guide

Second Edition

Valerie Aarne Grossman, MALS, BSN, NE-BC
Editor

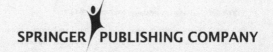

SPRINGER PUBLISHING COMPANY

Springer Publishing Company, LLC
11 West 42nd Street, New York, NY 10036
www.springerpub.com
connect.springerpub.com/

Acquisitions Editor: Rachel X. Landes
Compositor: Amnet Systems

ISBN: 978-0-8261-3929-0
ebook ISBN: 978-0-8261-3932-0
DOI: 10.1891/9780826139320

20 21 22 23 / 5 4 3 2 1

The author and the publisher of this Work have made every effort to use sources believed to be reliable to provide information that is accurate and compatible with the standards generally accepted at the time of publication. Because medical science is continually advancing, our knowledge base continues to expand. Therefore, as new information becomes available, changes in procedures become necessary. We recommend that the reader always consult current research and specific institutional policies before performing any clinical procedure or delivering any medication. The author and publisher shall not be liable for any special, consequential, or exemplary damages resulting, in whole or in part, from the readers' use of, or reliance on, the information contained in this book. The publisher has no responsibility for the persistence or accuracy of URLs for external or third-party Internet websites referred to in this publication and does not guarantee that any content on such websites is, or will remain, accurate or appropriate.

Library of Congress Cataloging-in-Publication Data
Names: Grossman, Valerie G. A., editor.
Title: Fast facts for the radiology nurse : an orientation and nursing care
  guide / Valerie Aarne Grossman, editor.
Other titles: Fast facts (Springer Publishing Company)
Description: Second edition. | New York, NY : Springer Publishing Company,
  LLC, [2020] | Series: Fast facts | Includes bibliographical references
  and index. |
Identifiers: LCCN 2020011128 (print) | LCCN 2020011129 (ebook) | ISBN
  9780826139290 (paperback) | ISBN 9780826139320 (ebook)
Subjects: MESH: Radiologic and Imaging Nursing | Nursing Care—methods
Classification: LCC RC78.7.D53 (print) | LCC RC78.7.D53 (ebook) | NLM WY
  167 | DDC 616.07/57—dc23
LC record available at https://lccn.loc.gov/2020011128
LC ebook record available at https://lccn.loc.gov/2020011129

Contact us to receive discount rates on bulk purchases.
We can also customize our books to meet your needs.
For more information please contact: sales@springerpub.com

Valerie Aarne Grossman: orcid.org/0000-0002-7648-7113

This book is dedicated to my family—John and Marie Aarne, Sarah and Steve Thyne, Nicole Grossman, and Josh Kaplan—who have believed in my writing and love for the nursing profession. While you may not have always understood my curiosity, tears, frustrations, unending beliefs, or sense of humor, you have always believed in "me." Thank you, guys; you have fulfilled my life in ways that no words can describe.

This book is also dedicated to "all others" who allowed me to matter in your lives. Your investment and belief in me have not been taken lightly. I am honored to receive what you have given me. I reflect often on the life journey I have been blessed with and recognize that today didn't happen without the help of many of you. Thank you.

Contents

Part I RADIOLOGY FOUNDATION

Part II NURSING ESSENTIALS

Part III RADIOLOGIC IMAGING MODALITIES: CT AND MRI

Part IV INTERVENTIONAL RADIOLOGY

Part V DIAGNOSTIC AND OTHER IMAGING MODALITIES

Part VI SPECIAL ISSUES IN RADIOLOGY NURSING

Part VII EMERGING AREAS OF RADIOLOGY NURSING

Contributors

Nana Ohene Baah, MD
Assistant Professor, Interventional Radiology
University of Rochester Medical Center
Rochester, New York

Edith Brous, JD, MS, MPH, BSN, RN
Nurse Attorney
New York, New York

Ana Davis, MSN, RN, CNL
Staff Nurse Medical Imaging
Highland Hospital (URMC affiliate)
Rochester, New York

John P. Deveikis, MD
John Hopkins All Children's Hospital
St. Petersburg, Florida

Susan Deveikis, BSN, RN
John Hopkins All Children's Hospital
St. Petersburg, Florida

Brooke Grandusky, BSN, RN, CRN
eRecord Analyst and Programmer
Department of Imaging Sciences
University of Rochester Medical Center
Rochester, New York

Lora K. (Ott) Hromadik, PhD, RN
Associate Professor
Department of Nursing and Allied Health Professions
Indiana University of Pennsylvania
Indiana, Pennsylvania

Velecia Marston, RN
Staff Nurse Medical Imaging
Highland Hospital (URMC affiliate)
Rochester, New York

Anna C. Montejano, DNP, RN, PHN, CEN
Associate Professor
Point Loma Nazarene University
San Diego, California

Jong Hee Oh, MS, RN, CNL, CRNI, VA-BC
Assistant Nurse Manager
Vascular Access Team, Medical Imaging
Highland Hospital (URMC affiliate)
Rochester, New York

Ashwani Kumar Sharma, MD, MBBS
Associate Professor, Department of Imaging Sciences
University of Rochester Medical Center
Rochester, New York

Lynn Sayre Visser, MSN, RN, PHN, CEN, CPEN
Nurse Author
Loomis, California

Cy Wakeman
President and Founder
Reality-Based Leadership
Elkhorn, Nebraska

Polly Gerber Zimmermann, MS, MBA, RN-BC, CEN, ONC FAEN
Associate Professor
North Park University
Chicago, Illinois

Reviewers

Meredith Addison, MSN, RN, CEN, FAEN
Staff Nurse
Emergency Department, Regional Hospital
Clinical Adjunct Faculty, School of Nursing, Indiana State University
Terre Haute, Indiana

Alona Anisimova, BSN, RN
Travel Staff Nurse
Stepdown Surgical Trauma
Virginia Commonwealth University Medical Center
Moseley, Virginia

Joop Breuer, RN, CEN, FAEN
Nurse Educator/Charge Nurse
Leiden University Medical Center
Leiden, Netherlands

Yvette Conyers, DNP, MS, RN, FNP-C, CTN-B
Assistant Professor of Community Health Nursing
Wegmans School of Nursing
St. John Fisher College
Rochester, New York

Anne L. von Fricken Coonrad, JD, MS, RN
Associate Court Attorney, Unified Court System
Albany, New York
Nursing Department Lecturer, SUNY Empire State College
Troy, New York

Teresa Coyne, BSN, RN, CEN
Clinical Coordinator
Memorial Hermann Katy Convenient Care Center
Katy, Texas

Cathy Crosby, MS, RN, CNL, CRN
Clinical Nurse Leader, Diagnostic Imaging Department
UR Medicine/Thompson Health
Canandaigua, New York

Amy Dooley, MS, RN, CPAN, CAPA
Clinical Educator
PACU, Ambulatory Surgery, Pre-operative Center
Lahey Hospital and Medical Center
Burlington, Massachusetts

Trevor Abela Fiorentino, PhD (Cov), RN
Lecturer in Emergency Nursing and Resuscitation
Faculty of Health Sciences
University of Malta
Msida, Malta

Amy Graham, MPH, BSN, RN
Staff Nurse
Norwalk Hospital
Norwalk, Connecticut

Darren M. Hernandez, BSN, RN
Clinical Resource Administrator
Highland Hospital (URMC affiliate)
Rochester, New York

Tommye Hinton, MSN, RN, CPHQ, NEA-BC
Principal, BrownePoints Leadership Development/Coaching Firm
Appraiser, ANCC Magnet Recognition Program
Detroit, Michigan

Renee Semonin Holleran, PhD, FNP-BC, CEN, CFRN, CTRN (retired), CCRN (emeritus), FAEN
FNP-BC Hope Clinic
Salt Lake City, Utah

Takashi Kitanosono, MD
President, Northfield International Inc.
Honolulu, Hawaii

Mary Catherine Marshall, RN, BAAN
Staff Nurse, Imaging Sciences
University of Rochester Medical Center
Rochester, New York

Joel M. Mueller, MSHA, RN
Clinical Team Manager, University of Rochester
Medical Center Home Care
Staff Nurse, Borg and Ide Imaging
Rochester, New York

Caroline Northrup, MS, RN-BC
Nurse Manager, West 4 Medical Surgical
Highland Hospital (affiliate of URMC)
Rochester, New York

Dr. Jonathan L. Portelli, PhD, MSc, BSc (Hons.)
Radiography Lecturer, Department of Radiography
Faculty of Health Sciences
University of Malta
Msida, Malta

Wende Ryan, RN
ICU Senior Staff Nurse
Wollongong Hospital
Port Kembla, New South Wales
Australia

Kenneth Scerri
Chairperson, The Maltese Emergency Nurses' Association
Staff Nurse, Emergency Department
Mater Dei Hospital
Msida, Malta

Mary Molly Shea, MSN, RN, SANE, LNC
Patient Safety Investigation Coordinator
Erie County Medical Center
Buffalo, New York

Nancy Shelton, BSN, RN, EMT-P
Staff Nurse, Emergency Department
Clinical Documentation Specialist
Ascension St. Vincent's Health System
Birmingham, Alabama

Mindy Sutherland, MBA, RT (R) (CT)
Lead Technologist (retired), CT Scan
Highland Hospital (URMC affiliate)
Rochester, New York

Sarah L. Thyne, MEd, BS
Special Education Teacher
Midlakes Middle School
Phelps-Clifton Springs Central School District
Clifton Springs, New York

Emily J. Timmreck, MSN, RN, ACNP
Clinical Education and Training Officer
Peace Corps
Washington, DC

Reviewers

Wendy Vassallo, BSc (Hons.) (Melit.), MSc (Edin.), RN
Registered Nurse, Mater Dei Hospital Emergency Department
Faculty of Health Science
University of Malta
Msida, Malta

Lynn Sayre Visser, MSN, RN, PHN, CEN, CPEN
Nurse Author
Loomis, California

Emily Winters, MS, RN-BC, NEA-BC
Nursing Professional Development Specialist
Department of Education
Highland Hospital (URMC affiliate)
Rochester, New York

Andrew Wong, MS, RN, AGACNP-BC, CEN, CPEN, CCRN-K
Clinical Impact Nurse Practitioner
Critical Care Medicine
Lenox Hill Hospital
Northwell Health System
New York, New York

Foreword

In the ever-changing environment of imaging nursing, *Fast Facts for the Radiology Nurse, Second Edition,* provides a quick and easy-to-use guide for the novice as well as the experienced radiology nurse. As technology improves the capabilities and reach of patient care in imaging medicine so do the demands for expert nursing care in radiology. From diagnostic, nuclear medicine, ultrasonography, magnetic resonance, computerized tomographic imaging, and interventional radiology, this book will provide a handy guide for all nursing care in the imaging environment.

Reflecting the most current guidelines and protocols, this second edition includes new chapters on Legal Issues Affecting Radiology, Strategies for Working With Difficult People, Safety and Quality in the Radiology Setting, and Emergency Management and Catastrophe Response. Fifty different interventional radiology procedures are covered including the importance of effective communication within the interventional radiology team.

Radiology nurses come from many areas, with diverse levels of experience but they all have one common goal—to deliver expert care in an imaging setting. This second edition of *Fast Facts for the Radiology Nurse* will give them a patient-centered, comprehensive, pocket-sized guide. It is a must have for every radiology department.

Donna Margiotta, BSN, RN, CRN
President-elect
Association of Radiologic Imaging Nursing

Foreword

Radiology departments have an ever-increasing need for highly skilled and competent radiology nurses to work in all the imaging modalities. Radiology nurses are important members of the radiology team, contributing to safe, effective, and quality patient care. Keeping informed on new diagnostic and therapeutic procedures is challenging for the experienced nurse and can be overwhelming for the nurse who is new to the imaging areas. This handbook serves as an important primer for nurses who are novices in the imaging areas and as a valuable reference for nurses with radiology experience who need fast, reliable information if working in a modality that is less familiar.

This second edition handbook offers information regarding the basic skills that a radiology nurse uses in everyday practice. Nurses draw from prior critical care, postanesthesia, and/or emergency nursing knowledge and assessment skills in radiology and also learn new skills specific to the imaging environment, including vascular access, hemostasis, infection control, physiological monitoring, and documentation. Additional updated information on sedation and analgesia includes medications in easy-to-read tables. New chapters in this second edition discuss legal issues, civility, disaster management, and leadership. These new topics are essential to the success of the nurse working in an imaging setting. Tables and figures enhance the chapters. "Fast Facts" boxes, which are located throughout the book, highlight key information.

An experienced radiology nurse clinician, nurse manager, and published author, Ms. Grossman, Editor, *Fast Facts for the Radiology Nurse*, has a passion for nursing and an inexhaustible commitment to elevate her chosen professional specialty of radiology nursing through advancing the literature for radiology nursing. These qualities have remained unchanged from the first edition. Ms. Grossman knows and understands what radiology nurses want and need to know to provide the best patient care and to be a member of a productive team. She has carefully chosen authors from a wide range of workplaces.

In summary, this handbook is a welcome addition to the resources for radiology nursing, which are few in number compared to other specialties. The handbook, which is in a pocket form, allows for easy reference, especially when the nurse may be traversing different modalities, for example, CT, MRI, or infrared, to provide bedside care. Nurses in other units, for example, medical–surgical or critical care, who care for radiology patients pre or post procedures will also appreciate the information in this handbook to improve patient care.

Kathleen A. Gross, MSN, RN-BC, CRN

Preface

Many nurses who enter the specialty areas of radiology nursing come from vastly different backgrounds of our profession. Over the years, I have worked with nurses who came to radiology from settings that include mental health, critical care, medical–surgical, ambulatory, surgical services, groups homes . . . the list is endless. They all bring vast and unique experiential knowledge with them to the radiology setting. Becoming a radiology nurse is an excellent example of Benner's nursing theory of novice to expert. These nurses were experts in their prior positions and are suddenly in an environment that may be so very foreign to them; they will have to begin their acquisition of knowledge and proficiency from a very uncomfortable place of being a beginner again. The journey is worth the effort: Radiology nurses will be the first to tell others that a *bad day in radiology is often better than the best day on the floors*. It just is!

Learning to be a radiology nurse takes us out of the nursing lead environment and puts us in departments that were started with radiologists and technologists. Some nurses never find comfort in this arrangement (and leave), and others work to figure it out. The focus of any imaging arena is to obtain great images for the radiologist to read so the ordering provider can receive the answers they are seeking in the care and diagnosis of their patient. In the interventional radiology suite, the patient may need a procedure that is either diagnostic or therapeutic, and again, this is performed by a physician and a technologist at the request of the ordering provider. Nurses who enter this specialty must be ready to be flexible and invest in their own learning pathway.

Many sources exist to assist the nurse in this acquisition of knowledge. The *Journal of Radiology Nursing* diligently works to provide nurses with up-to-date information regarding our focus of practice. The Association for Radiology and Imaging Nursing (ARIN) has developed a core curriculum from the knowledge of a vast nursing team of volunteers. We utilize information from the American College of Radiology (ACR), the Society of Interventional Radiology (SIR), and a number of other organizations to enhance our knowledge.

This next edition of *Fast Facts for the Radiology Nurse* was written to further serve the needs of nurses in a variety of radiology settings. Basic information such as personal accountability, vascular access, and contrast safety is essential for any radiology nurse. Strategies and essential information needed when caring for the diverse patient population who come to us with their complex health issues (physical and emotional) are included in a streamlined fashion. Every patient can present a uniquely challenging situation for the radiology nurse, and there are strategies included to assist the nurse in providing them with safe care.

Radiology departments are made up of a variety of different services. This book includes the knowledge and expertise of 43 contributors and reviewers from around the world, with the common goal of providing the reader with basic information that will help the nurse jump feet-first into the clinical setting of radiology nursing!

Valerie Aarne Grossman

Acknowledgments

This book could not have happened if it were not for the passion, perseverance, and belief in the "frontline nurse" that Elizabeth Nieginski possesses. Elizabeth is an award-winning editor who is currently the publisher for nursing with Springer Publishing Company. Her dedication to not only quality publications but to the endless support of their authors is unmatched. She has devoted her life to nursing publications, and for that, we are all thankful.

I am grateful to the team of contributors (14) and reviewers (29) from around the world who came together and volunteered their time and expertise to the second edition of this book. It takes team members, with high moral standards, who believe in the very best patient care to make a difference. Thank you for believing in this project!

I

Radiology Foundation

1

Introduction to Radiology Nursing and Radiation Safety

Valerie Aarne Grossman

Radiology nursing is an emerging specialty area that requires a variety of skills. Gaining expertise will take time and patience along with ongoing professional development. Radiation safety is essential for all members of a radiology team as well as patients being cared for.

In this chapter, you will discover:

1. The complexity of radiology nursing
2. Importance of collaboration
3. Safe radiation practices

The world of radiology is changing very quickly. Not too long ago, the only caregivers in any given radiology department were the radiologist and the licensed technologist. Now, there may be a complex team of transporters, unlicensed assistive personnel, nurses, technologists, advanced practice providers as well as the radiologists! As the complexity of healthcare grows, so too does imaging ability. Different modalities, technologies, and skill levels must all work in harmony to provide precision images for the radiologist, who will ultimately provide insight into a patient's condition for the ordering provider. Decreasing reimbursement, increasing regulation, increasing sophistication, and increasing census, combined with the different practice styles and needs of the radiology modalities, can lead to a very confusing nursing environment that is continually changing and ever challenging (Donnelly, Dickerson, Goodfriend, & Muething, 2010).

Nursing is quickly gaining a greater presence in radiology settings. The increasing complexity of procedures within the modalities as well as patients with more complex healthcare issues require the expertise of motivated nursing professionals. Radiology nurses must be proactive, patient-focused, and able to work with a diverse team of individuals. Often, the nurses in radiology are breaking new ground, discovering new patient care issues, and amending practice to meet new regulations. A radiology nurse must be able to care for the widest range of patients (much like a nurse in the ED) from pediatric to geriatric, from trauma to oncology, from self-care patients to total care patients . . . there is no *routine patient* in an imaging department.

The risk of potential error is monumental. Wrong patient, wrong order, wrong study, wrong laterality, satisfaction of search (missing a key finding on the image) . . . every patient has so many individual components of each study; just one wrong step can severely affect the outcome of the imaging study for that patient (Ridley, 2017).

Beyond that, a radiology nurse must remember that there is a person behind each and every image . . . someone with a life that matters, a story worth sharing. In the chaos of a normal workday, it can sometimes be easy for the nurse to forget how the patient sees their visit to radiology: *Will this scan show there is a tumor? Will this ultrasound show that I'm pregnant? Can this interventional radiology (IR) procedure stop the bleeding?* Our radiology environment is "normal" for us but to our patients who trust us with their lives, it may be foreign and scary. It is our role as professionals to guide each patient through their time with us in radiology and treat them with dignity and respect.

Fast Facts

Refrain from the use of personal electronic devices while in the clinical area. This is an infection control risk and causes our patients/visitors to misperceive where our attention is focused.

RADIATION SAFETY

Today's advancing medical imaging arenas provide physicians with state-of-the-art technology to see within a body through diagnostic imaging tools. Yet, that ability comes with a degree of risk. The radiology team must protect not only the patient but also themselves in this environment. Some simple rules should be followed 100% of the time when working with radiation in the areas of CT scan, PET scan, interventional radiology, x-ray, nuclear medicine, mammography, cardiac catheter lab, operating room with a C-arm, or any number of other settings.

The very common term ALARA (as low as reasonably achievable) refers to the recommendation that the technologist use the lowest amount of radiation possible to achieve the image the radiologist needs. This is not a "one-step" process, as it may involve utilizing other modalities that do not use radiation (ultrasound or MRI), or if the best study for the patient uses radiation, then the team must consider increasing the distance from the source of radiation, decreasing the time of exposure to radiation, and using the appropriate shielding for the patient or staff.

- **Time**
  - Decreasing the amount of exposure time will automatically decrease the dose of radiation to the patient and the provider.
  - Thorough planning of the image or the procedure will be necessary with streamlined workflow, precise protocols, and operational expertise of the equipment and/or radioactive material by the technologist.
- **Distance**
  - Increasing the distance from the source of radiation will decrease the exposure dose.
- **Shielding**
  - Using the appropriate type of shielding will protect the individual from exposure. A variety of products are available including lead aprons, lead shielding stands, goggles, thyroid shields, and sterile drapes that cover the patients during procedures (Conner & Blanchard, 2011).

Fast Facts

With mounting concerns about the carcinogenic effects of imaging techniques, all imaging providers need to keep as a priority the safety of staff and patients through utilization of the lowest dose possible for the imaging outcome desired as well as ALARA (Oakley, Ehsani, & Harrison, 2019).

UNANTICIPATED ADVERSE EVENTS

All staff in any imaging environment need to strive for complete safety of our patients. From radiation safety to meticulous care of our most critically unstable patients, the imaging team must work in concert to provide the highest quality and the safest of patient care. Patients may be at great risk for falls, allergic reactions, intravenous (IV) extravasations, blood transfusion reactions, clinical decompensation, behavioral outbursts . . . the list goes on. All staff must maintain a heightened attention to our patients and be ready to react to any situation that may occur.

Ensuring patient safety is as essential as maintaining the safety of our team members. Occupational exposures or incidents place our colleagues in jeopardy and should be addressed just as seriously as any adverse patient event. With the increasing opioid crisis and the deterioration of society's ability to maintain emotional self-control, our staff members are at risk of workplace injury more now than ever before (Chipidza, Wallwork, Adams, & Stern, 2016).

Event reporting maintains safety in the radiology setting. Documenting "near misses" and "good catches" are just as important as documenting the most serious of events. These event reports can assist in the organization's ability to create safer practices going forward (Siewert, Swedeen, Brook, Eisenberg, & Hockman, 2018). An environment of "Just Culture" should exist, which promotes an open reporting environment, takes the focus away from the event being linked to a specific person, and analyzes the process by which an error occurred (Boysen, 2013).

Fast Facts

All imaging arenas should promote a *Just Culture* for accurate reporting and evaluation of all adverse events to occur.

For situations of a more serious nature, an organization may conduct a root cause analysis (RCA) to allow a team to evaluate the event, identify steps of concern, and create recommendations for the future. Crucial to the success of an RCA are three elements:

1. Specific details of the adverse event
2. Analysis of the event steps and recommendations to prevent them from happening in the future

3. Development of new process steps along with education of the team. Follow-up steps for any RCA should also include:

- Counseling for the staff involved, as employees may suffer emotional trauma from any clinical error or adverse event affecting their patient
- Chart reviews to assess the new process instituted to verify the change in practice, and if additional changes should occur, these will guard against the adverse event from recurring in the future (Brook, Kruskal, Eisenberg, & Larson, 2015)

References

Boysen, P. (2013). Just culture: A foundation for balanced accountability and patient safety. *The Ochsner Journal, 13*(3), 400–406.

Brook, O., Kruskal, J., Eisenberg, R., & Larson, D. (2015). Root cause analysis: Learning from adverse safety events. *RadioGraphics, 35*(6), 1655–1667. doi:10.1148/rg.2015150067

Chipidza, F., Wallwork, R. S., Adams, T. N., & Stern, T. A. (2016). Evaluation and treatment of the angry patient. *The Primary Care Companion for CNS Disorders, 18*(3), 10.4088/PCC.16f01951. doi:10.4088/PCC.16f01951

Conner, R., & Blanchard, J. (2011) Recommended practices for reducing radiological exposure in the perioperative practice setting. *Perioperative Standards and Recommended Practices, 2011*, 251–261.

Donnelly, L., Dickerson, J., Goodfriend, M., & Muething, S. (2010). Improving patient safety in radiology. *American Journal of Roentgenology, 194*, 1183–1187.

Oakley, P. A., Ehsani, N. N., & Harrison, D. E. (2019). The Scoliosis Quandary: Are radiation exposures from repeated X-rays harmful? *Dose-Response, 17*(2), 1559325819852810. doi:10.1177/1559325819852810

Ridley, E. (2017). How can radiology departments ensure patient safety? *AuntMinnie.com*. Retrieved from https://www.auntminnie.com/index .aspx?sec=prtf&sub=def&pag=dis&itemId=116697&printpage=true&fse c=rca&fsub=ecr_2017

Siewert, B., Swedeen, S., Brook, O., Eisenberg, R., & Hockman, M. (2018). Barriers to safety event reporting in an Academic Radiology Department: Authority gradients and other human factors. *Radiology, 288*(3), 693–698. doi:10.1148/radiol.2018171625

2

Teamwork Essentials

Polly Gerber Zimmermann

The public expects healthcare providers to be professional in all that they do while providing the safest precision patient care possible. Those who work within a healthcare setting recognize some colleagues are difficult to work with and, at times, unprofessional. Studies have shown poor communication and a weak team can lead to increased errors in a healthcare setting. Regulatory agencies set standards for organizations to follow to maintain safer environments for the patients they care for.

In this chapter, you will discover:

1. How to promote "team"
2. How to set boundaries with coworkers
3. How to handle escalating behavior

TEAMWORK

"There is no 'i' in team" is a common, but often impotent, phrase. To create a group that wants the same goals, there must be an atmosphere that promotes comfort, camaraderie, and security with coworkers who are comfortable speaking up while supporting patient safety and quality care.

Building Teamwork

- Communicate reasons to enhance pride and tradition within the department.
    - People do not worry about being fired as much as falling into disfavor or not belonging to the group.
- Compliment in public; criticize in private.
    - Identify at least one thing for each department member that the person does well and mention it in front of others.
- Look for an opportunity to tell another person's boss how well they did: it *will* get back to them.
- Find something outside of work that is important to each person in the department.
    - Regularly discuss that topic with them so that your only interaction is not work. Common subjects include children/ grandchildren, hobbies, or vacation.
- Consider a department meeting where universal expectations and code of conduct are identified, agreed upon, and posted.
    - Hold everyone to the same level of accountability.

Dealing With Change: The One Constant in Life Is Change

- Involve the affected individuals when determining change.
- Appeal to higher core, common values, such as "safe patient care," "quality," or "effectiveness."
    - Who would ever publicly admit that they do not care about those motivators?
- Communicate the reason for the change.
    - Whenever possible, ask frontline staff for their opinions and ideas.
- Work privately to build a supportive consensus before any public presentation.
    - Start with the early adaptors.
- Know best practices and cite them as it shows what is possible.
- Cite a higher authority when asking for change or agreement. Sources can include:
    - Professional association recommendations
    - A published article
    - A senior administrator
    - What other hospitals are doing in the local area
    - Regulations
    - Lawsuits

BULLYING IN HEALTHCARE

"Bullying" or "disruptive behavior" is not acceptable in healthcare either by staff or patients/families. Not only is disruptive behavior demoralizing, but it also affects the quality of care. In one study, 76% of respondents reported that disruptive behaviors were linked to adverse events, such as medical errors (71%) and patient mortality (27%) (Roche, Diers, Duffield, & Catling-Paull, 2010). Healthcare organizations have paid closer attention to difficult behaviors since The Joint Commission's 2008 development of a leadership standard regarding "behaviors that undermine a culture of safety" (Wyatt, 2013). According to a survey conducted by the Institute for Safe Medication Practices (ISMP), of the 4,884 respondents considering their previous year of practice, it was reported: 77% encountered reluctance/refusal of a colleague to answer a question or return a phone call; 68% encountered condescending or demeaning insults; and 69% encountered having someone hang up the phone on them (ISMP, 2013).

Fast Facts

- Say something positive as the first thing you say to everyone every day.
- Establish behavioral policies and expectations, such as chain of command and/or zero tolerance.
- Focus on improving the process rather than the person.

Dealing With "Disruptive" Healthcare Providers

Verbal and Nonverbal Abuse

Signs
- Sighing, rolling eyes
- Abrupt response/walking away while the other professional is talking
- Sarcasm, snide remarks
- Talking behind back
- Undermining/withholding information
- Negative comments about colleagues or leaders
- Refusal to answer questions
- Reluctance to follow safety practices or work collaboratively

Responsive Behaviors

- Deal with the action and request what you expect. Practice these phrases to use, especially if new to the department:
  - "I sense that there may be something you wanted to say to me. It's okay to speak directly to me."
  - "The individuals I learn the most from are clearer in their directions and feedback. Is there some way we can structure this type of situation?"
  - "When something happens that is 'different' or 'contrary' to what I thought or understood, it leaves me with questions. Help me understand how this situation may have happened."
  - "It is my understanding that there was more information available regarding this situation, and I believe if I had known that, it would affect how I learn."
- Use assertive communication with "I" statements that address behaviors (not personality).
  - "I've noticed _____."
  - "When you do_____, I feel _____."
  - "I need you to _____."
- Use TeamSTEPPS Advocacy and Assertion (DHHS, 2019) to outline the steps to take when you are Concerned, Uncomfortable, or recognize a Safety concern (CUS) about what is currently happening.
  - Make an opening.
  - State the concern.
  - Offer a corrective action in a firm and respectful manner.
  - Obtain an agreement.
  - If ignored, *repeat the request a second time*. If not satisfied, then take stronger action such as activating the chain of command.

Fast Facts

Up to 80% of the time, nurses deal with difficulties by avoidance. Besides the stress of unresolved conflict, failing to address inappropriate behaviors creates a culture where deviancy is "normalized."

Specific Person Abuse

Signs

- Specific negative language or behavior directed toward an individual, including sexual harassment
- Screaming, throwing things, profanity
- Hanging up the telephone prior to the conclusion of the conversation

Responsive Behaviors

- Tell the person to stop.
- Tell the person the discussion must be taken private. Turn around and walk away.
- "Code White/Code Pink": All staff members surround a verbally attacked staff member. They stand silent with arms crossed and stare at the disruptive individual who usually stops the offending behavior.
  - An ounce of prevention is worth a pound of cure when dealing with upset patients or family members. Set a positive tone from the first contact.

Patient/Family General Hints

- Look up and beam when greeting people (keep the area over your heart open).
- Consider a scripted apology ("I'm sorry you had to wait") anytime you do not immediately take the patient in.
- Compliment parents on their children (all parents think their children are good looking and above average!)
- Remark to a child about "how big" they are.
- Do not interrupt the person when he or she is speaking to you.
  - The average healthcare provider interrupts 23 seconds into the patient's statement.

Dealing With "Disruptive Patients/Families"

Disruptive behavior is on a continuum. Recognize escalation and intervene appropriately.

First Stage: Challenging the Provider

Signs

- Voice changes tone, volume, or cadence from normal conversation.
- Body language changes, such as muscle tenseness, anger expression, or leaning forward.

De-escalation Responses

- Ignore challenges to the nurse's qualifications or actions; redirect to the issue at hand to avoid a power struggle.
- Do not quote authoritative rules.
  - "You can't act like that! This is a hospital" rarely changes behavior.
- Let the person vent and do not deny the complaint to "deflate" the emotion.
- Acknowledge the person's emotions ("I can see you are angry") so the person feels validated.

- Use the person's name often as it grabs the rational part of the brain.
- Consider a "blameless apology."
  - "I am sorry you had a problem."
  - Seek to move forward: "What can we do now to get you the care you need?"

Second Stage: Refusal and Noncompliance

Signs

- Becomes more argumentative and challenging

De-escalation Responses

- Set limits and specifically name unacceptable behavior (threatening, swearing).
  - "I felt put down by your sarcastic comment about ___. I treat you in a respectful manner and I need you to do the same when you interact with me."
- Consider a verbal contract to control behavior
  - "Can you do ___ while I do ___?"
- Focus on concrete needs (cup of coffee, cell phone charger, meal, etc.)

Third Stage: Emotional Release

Signs

- Outburst, with higher intensity
- Loss of rational thought

De-escalation Responses

- Remove from public arena.
- Restate what the person is saying.
- Share your emotional response ("Now you are scaring me"). It may make them realize they are losing control.
- Give undivided attendance.

Fourth Stage: Intimidation

Signs

- Verbal or nonverbal threats.
- You feel frightened in your gut: Trust yourself.

De-escalation Responses

- Stand one-leg length away, and give personal space.
- Always have an exit available.
- Get assistance (security, panic button).

Tension Reduction

Once the environment is controlled, reassure individuals that they will receive quality care.

De-Escalation Resources

Crisis Prevention Institute: www.crisisprevention.com
Ten Critical De-escalation Skills: www.populararticles.com/article45613.html

References

Institute for Safe Medication Practices. (2013, October 3). Unresolved disrespectful behavior in healthcare—Practitioners speak up again (Part 1). *ISMP Medical Safety Alert.* Retrieved from https://www.ismp.org/resources/unresolved-disrespectful-behavior-healthcare-practitioners-speak-again-part-i

Roche, M., Diers, D., Duffield, C., & Catling-Paull, C. (2010). Violence towards nurses, the work environment, and patient outcomes. *Journal of Nursing Scholarship, 24*(1), 13–22. doi:10.1111/j.1547-5069.2009.01321.x

U.S. Department of Health and Human Services. (2019). TeamSTEPPS. *Agency for Healthcare Research and Quality.* Retrieved from https://www.ahrq.gov/teamstepps/instructor/essentials/igessentials.html

Wyatt, R. (2013). Revisiting disruptive and inappropriate behavior: Five years after standards introduced. *The Joint Commission High Reliability Healthcare: Center for Transforming Healthcare Leaders.* Retrieved from https://www.jointcommission.org/jc_physician_blog/revisiting_disruptive_and_inappropriate_behavior/

3

Five Ways to Modernize Your Leadership and Get Rid of the Drama

Cy Wakeman

Leadership training is currently reinforcing bad behaviors, not fixing them. We are spending more and more time and more and more money on training boot camps, yet things are not getting better. So, what is the problem? In this chapter, I break down five key ways we need to change our leadership philosophies. These are easy, actionable things you can do today.

In this chapter, you will discover:

1. How to decrease workplace drama
2. How to evaluate leadership styles
3. The difference between sympathy and empathy

I am Cy Wakeman, and I am a thought leader in human resources and leadership and a drama researcher. In this chapter, I show you five ways you absolutely need to update your leadership philosophy. Many people do not even realize traditional leadership philosophies, the ones you have likely been taught and the ones you have been practicing, do not help. They actually hurt. They are fueling drama at work, and they are creating entitlement.

The work experience is so full of drama, and it is seen as a normal cost of doing business. But drama is both avoidable and has a real, negative financial impact. Drama leads to lost productivity, peace, and happiness. Have you noticed? More than visible squabbles and emotional outbursts at work, drama also includes ego-based resistance to change, employee disengagement, and lack of alignment to strategic initiatives (Wakeman, 2010).

While there is no lack of leadership and human resource (HR) training, tools, and techniques, current strategies have not dealt with the root causes of drama (what I call emotional waste). The 2.5 hours per employee per day that workplaces spend on drama adds up to *816 hours per year* (Wakeman, 2017). Imagine what could be recaptured and created instead.

#1: STOP BLAMING YOUR CIRCUMSTANCES

Your circumstances are not the reasons you cannot succeed, and they are not the reasons your team cannot succeed. Yet, when people complain about what is not working, tattle on other teams not doing their fair share, or tell you about something in their reality that makes it tough for them to do their jobs, like most leaders, you may be tempted to jump to fix these problems for them. But when you do, you leave your team believing the reason they cannot succeed is their circumstances, *when, in fact, their reality and their circumstances are not the reasons they cannot succeed, but rather they are the reality in which they must succeed.*

Attempting to "fix" circumstances not only leads a team to believe their circumstances are an excuse but also robs them of their own development. When people come to you, your job is not to overmanage and fix things. Your job is to lead. Stop overmanaging and start leading. Instead, when people come to you and you are tempted to go fix the situation, stop and instead focus on growing, coaching, and developing the person in front of you. When people come to you complaining about adverse circumstances or tattling on other teams, shift their focus to themselves.

How does a leader begin to facilitate introspection and self-reflection that will spur personal growth and development? It is not as difficult as you may imagine. I love having a list of great questions ready when I give feedback. Here are some of my favorites:

- What do you know for sure?
- What could you do next to add value?
- How can you help?
- What would look great right now?
- What did you do that hindered progress or success? What helped?
- If you did not have the story you are telling yourself right now, who would you be?
- How is that working for you?

Fast Facts

Your circumstances are not the reasons you cannot succeed; they are the reality in which you must succeed.

#2 MANAGE ENERGY, NOT PEOPLE

Great leaders need to focus on managing the energy of the situation rather than the people in the room. In my research, I look at where energy is going during meetings. In over 90% of the meetings I observed, the energy was focused on *"Why we couldn't,"* *"Why we shouldn't have to,"* and *"Why that idea won't work."* And the leaders went along with it! They were problem-solving about how to get people's buy-in rather than how to deliver what the organization needed.

In your future meetings and your interactions with people, move the energy away from *"Why we can't"* to *"How we could,"* and from *"Why we shouldn't have to"* to *"How we can deliver exquisitely."* Make sure that you are using empathy, not sympathy. *Sympathy* is hearing you are in pain and validating your victim mindset; the reason you are in pain is your circumstances or other people, things outside yourself. What does this sound like in real life? When someone comes in to complain, I listen and sympathize. I start to agree with you and collude with you, leaving you to believe we are in this situation because of somebody else.

Empathy is acknowledging I see you struggling right now, but it is followed by a call to greatness. I see you are suffering, so let us talk about what we need to do to mitigate the risks you are concerned about and move forward.

All too often, I see leaders roll things out with sympathy instead of empathy. Have you ever rolled out a new strategy or change by starting with an apology? Here is what that sounds like:

> *"I'm so sorry. I know you're all so busy. I hate to bring another thing onto your plate, but I've been instructed that this is a have-to, it's mandatory. So, if you, out of the goodness of your heart, can just please, please, please get on board and do your best."*

Let us stop right there. You have just taught people that buy-in is optional. In contrast, here is what empathy looks like:

> *"I have some new information that we need to deliver on, and it's going to involve changing our business processes. So, I'm going to let you know*

what I know, and then we're going to go around the table, and we're going to focus on what we need to do to make this change least disruptive. Now let's talk about how we can do this. What are your ideas?"

Leading with empathy rather than sympathy takes the energy of the meeting away from *"why we shouldn't have to"* or *"why it's a dumb idea"* and puts the focus of your team on creatively solving the problem within current constraints and resources.

Fast Facts

Too many leaders use sympathy to connect with employees when they should use empathy and a call to greatness.

#3 SUFFERING IS COMPLETELY OPTIONAL (AND USUALLY SELF-IMPOSED)

I am not talking about suffering from a medical sense. I am talking about the suffering we cause for ourselves when we believe all our thinking. Your suffering and the suffering of your team are not coming from their circumstances or reality. It actually comes from the story we make up about our reality. Your suffering is optional. *There are two ways to go through today: with joy or misery, your choice.* As a leader, it is your job to help your team separate out suffering from reality. If you see your team hurting, that is an indication of where they need to grow next.

As an example, I worked on a team where we had to move multiple times in a short period of time. The team would often come to me very frustrated. They believed the reason they were suffering was all the moving, but that was not the case. The reason they were suffering was they had not yet learned to get mobile. That hurt more than the fact that we had to move. If our reality is that we move a lot, how can we make it so that we can be very fast in our moving and not have any pain around it? How can we grow in our own mobility?

Fast Facts

There are two ways to go through today: with joy or misery, your choice.

#4 WORK WITH THE WILLING

I cannot tell you the number of emails and calls I get where people want to get somebody who is chronically resistant on board and *my best piece of advice is to work with the willing.* All too often, we try to bring along resistant people by falling back on conventional change-management techniques that attempt to outwit the resistance and cajole them into buy-in and participation with extra bouts of awareness and encouragement. But there is a prerequisite to making behavioral change work: willingness (Wakeman, 2013).

Often leaders use hope as a strategy with employees who have told them by their actions that they are unwilling. Instead of believing their employees' actions, these leaders delegate work around them and dream they will get willing and on board. When that strategy fails, leaders justify their actions with, *"Well, we have to deal with this behavior because there's a talent shortage out there."*

On average, a leader will spend 80 extra hours a year thinking about and working with a single person who is in a chronic state of resistance (Wakeman, 1992). The average return on this hefty investment is, at most, 3%. Bottom line: Your odds of changing someone in resistance are close to zero. If you focus on those in resistance, you are paying them to bully you and to critique and sabotage your plans. The worst part is the other people you lead will notice, and they will want attention too.

Wake-up call. *Your job as a leader is to make people aware of the business realities, opportunities, and challenges and to call people up to greatness.* Remember that *buy-in is not optional. Buy in is a verb.* Employees need to remember this, too. They need to go first and buy into the strategic direction of the team and company. Too many times we put the responsibility on the leader to get somebody bought in, but the individual's willingness is their business. You can only work with the willing.

The best strategy I have found when you are working with somebody who is resistant or withholding buy-in is to test their willingness. These "are you willing" questions sound like this:

- Now that you are aware of what is needed, what is your level of willingness to get skilled in this area as a professional?
- On a scale of 1 to 10, where do you think you are? And if the rating is low, what is your plan to get more willing?
- If you are not on board, what is your plan to transition out of the organization?
- How can you show me that you are willing?

Willingness is more than getting their plan turned into you; it is the true level of real buy-in action. If they are not willing, it is game over and the next gesture of help is to lovingly assist them in their transition out of the organization to pursuits more aligned with their goals.

There are really only two options: to stay in joy or leave in peace. I have worked with a lot of people who thought there was a third option to stay and hate, to stay and sabotage, to stay and not get on board until, I as a leader, helped them see reality. There is no third option.

#5: QUESTION CONVENTIONAL LEADERSHIP PHILOSOPHIES

I started my career as a therapist. When I was promoted to my first leadership position, I was shocked at the content in my leadership-development courses that ran counter to the evidence-based learning I was accustomed to in psychology. I actually made my career out of questioning conventional wisdom most people have just accepted.

Here is an example I heard over and over again: Change is hard. But I found in my research that *change is only hard for the unready.* Change by itself is not hard; what makes it hard is whether or not you are ready for it.

Let us say that you have two great employees; one has refused to upgrade to a smartphone. They have the same flip phone they have owned since high school. The other employee upgrades their technology as often as possible to ensure they have access to all the tools and resources that a great smartphone can provide. Now the change comes, and you give each of them a new smartphone. Is change equally hard for them? No! Change is only hard for the unready—for the employee with the flip phone.

To break the scenario down, the employee who has always upgraded takes the new smartphone and their attitude toward you is one of gratitude. They are excited for their new smartphone. They go to the cloud, get their stuff, and are ready to go in about 5 minutes. The employee who has the flip phone is curled up in the fetal position. You have to hold a change initiative and training class to get them up to date. But see, it is not the change that was hard. This employee just was not ready for the change.

There are so many simple things you are saying on a daily basis, like, *"Change is hard,"* or *"There's too much change,"* that I want you to stop and question. When you find team members are struggling with change, take it as a sign to check one of three areas:

1. Their current skillset
2. Their current mindset
3. Their current approach

It is time to admit that the traditional leadership techniques we have been taught are not working and, in fact, are causing more drama and entitlement in our workplace than ever. If you want to learn about how to get rid of the drama in your organization and get back to producing results, follow me on social media and YouTube @CyWakeman and subscribe to my weekly podcast (https://CyWakeman.lnk.to/NoEgo), where I share my best tips and techniques on restoring sanity to the workplace.

Fast Facts

Change itself is not hard; what makes it hard is whether you are ready for it or not.

References

Wakeman, C. (1992). *Resistant employees' drain on management resources.* Omaha, NE: Clarkson College Graduate Program.

Wakeman, C. (2010). *Reality-based leadership: Ditch the drama, restore sanity to the workplace, and turn excuses into results.* San Francisco, CA: Jossey-Bass.

Wakeman, C. (2013). *Reality-based rules of the workplace: Know what boosts your value, kills your chances, and will make you happier.* San Francisco, CA: Jossey-Bass.

Wakeman, C. (2017). *No ego: How leaders can cut the cost of workplace drama, end entitlement, and drive big results.* New York, NY: St. Martin's Press.

4

Recent Developments in Nursing Care

Polly Gerber Zimmermann

Depending on how "seasoned" a nurse is, the memory trail of past outdated practices can be quite long. There are social-environmental changes such as nursing caps. More important are the advances in quality and safety in providing healthcare. Who can remember the days of

- caregiving without gloves (it would offend the patient),
- milking chest tubes,
- humidifiers with standing water in patients' rooms,
- venous cutdowns (instead of peripherally inserted central catheter [PICC] lines), or
- checking a patient's glucose level with tablets and urine in a test tube instead of blood?

In this chapter, you will discover:

1. New twists to old skills
2. The association between opioid sedation and obstructive sleep apnea (OSA)
3. Updated safety actions

OPIOID-INDUCED SEDATION AND RESPIRATORY DEPRESSION/OSA

It is estimated that at least 9% of women and 24% of men have OSA; yet as many as 80% go undiagnosed. The classic risk factors for OSA are represented in the mnemonic *Stop Bang*:

Stop
- History of **S**noring loudly
- History of feeling **T**ired, fatigued, or sleepy during the day
- **O**bserved stop breathing during sleep
- History of past or current treatment for high blood **P**ressure (Chung et al., 2008)

Bang
- **B**MI > 35 (normal is 18.5–24.9; e.g., more than 10% over ideal)
- **A**ge > 50 years
- **N**eck circumference > 17 inches (40 cm)
- **G**ender: male

A patient with OSA is at increased risk for opioid-induced respiratory depression from narcotics or sedating medications. The body's response to the accumulating carbon dioxide is dulled, and the body cannot arouse itself to breathe. Monitoring for OSA includes noting loud snoring as that indicates obstruction: Normal respirations are quiet and effortless. Raise the head of the bed, if possible, to lessen the tongue falling back.

Monitor for excess sedation because sedation precedes respiratory depression. (Note: OSA does not cause respiratory distress.) The Pasero Opioid-Induced Sedation Scale (POSS) is a good tool to evaluate a patient's sedation. A patient unintentionally falling asleep while talking to you is at risk for respiratory depression.

The desired "normal" pulse oximetry for a healthy patient is 95% to 100%. A pulse oximeter reading of 90% is only equal to a 60 PaO_2. Remember the reversal agent for narcotics; naloxone (Narcan) has a shorter half-life than narcotics (45–90 minutes vs. up to 7 hours for a narcotic). It is possible for the patient to have a repeat apnea episode. Methadone (now being used for severe chronic pain) is 7.5 times the strength of morphine and has a half-life of up to 60 hours.

Fast Facts

Up to 80% of individuals with OSA go undiagnosed.

PROPER SPINAL PRECAUTIONS

Potential spinal cord injuries should have minimal movement. When patient movement is necessary, it is essential to do it properly. This includes:

- Do not use a "lift sheet"; it allows sagging.
- Use a minimum of three people to move the patient.
- Secure the head and torso. Using a cervical collar alone does not immobilize the cervical spine. Immobilization of the head and torso prevents flexion, extension, rotation, and lateral movement.
- Minimize the use of "logrolling." Using a scoop stretcher for movement instead can reduce overall cumulative motion to an unstable spine by 50%. Logrolling has been shown to produce significantly greater motion in the unstable cervical spine compared to other methods. This is because patient variances in dimensions make it difficult to maintain spinal alignment and proper logrolling requires excellent staff coordination/timing (ENA 2015 Trauma Committee, 2016).

Fast Facts

A minimum of three people must assist with the movement of a patient with spinal precautions.

MANAGEMENT OF NASOGASTRIC TUBES

- A blind insertion of a nasogastric tube must be verified with an x-ray before its initial use to instill fluid/medication. After that, placement can be verified by pH, not by listening to air gurgling (Bankhead et al., 2009).
- It is no longer necessary to hold the feeding if lowering the head of the bed for a short time just for repositioning or routine care. (The feeding is stopped for prolonged procedures.)

NEW DEFINITION FOR HYPERTENSION

As of November 2017, hypertension is defined as 130/80 (instead of 140/90) per the American College of Cardiology and American Heart Association.

NO ROUTINE OXYGEN APPLICATION FOR ACUTE MYOCARDIAL INFARCTION PATIENTS

Automatic use of oxygen for nonhypoxic patients with acute myocardial infarction (AMI) has been questioned as far back as 2004 because of the lack of a discernible benefit. A 2015 study found significantly higher morbidity with liberal use of supplemental oxygen in nonhypoxic AMI patients. In 2017, the European Society of Cardiology cited the lack of clear evidence for benefit and evidence for potential harm in their recommendation against routine use of supplemental oxygen for patients who are not hypoxic (e.g., $SpO_2 \geq 90\%$). The recommendation for AMI or stroke is to not initiate oxygen if the SpO_2 is $\geq 93\%$.

An April 2018 meta-analysis of 25 randomized trials showed significantly higher mortality with liberal use of supplemental oxygen in acutely ill patients compared with conservative oxygen use. The negative effects are hypothesized to be related to the oxygen acting as a free radical (Siemieniuk et al., 2018). There may be a lag for practice to catch up: One study found that 96% of surveyed physicians administered oxygen for all AMI patients (Chen & Lim, 2018).

TREATING VITAMIN DEFICIENCIES IN SEPSIS

Besides the timely administration of aggressive intravenous (IV) fluids and antibiotics, the new focus in sepsis management is looking at metabolic factors.

- Vitamin C levels drop in sepsis, and its deficiency is associated with multiple organ failure and death. Vitamin C is needed for catecholamine production, and administration resulted in less mortality.
- Thiamine deficiency was found in one-third of patients with sepsis. A 2018 study found its use reduces lactate and mortality.
- Adding hydrocortisone worked synergistically with vitamin C and improved sensitivity.

qSOFA FROM THE SEPSIS-3

A new focus is looking to be more precise and specific in sepsis criteria, especially related to affecting the body's organs. Lactate is now part of the early diagnostic criteria (Lester, Hartjes, & Bennett, 2018). The quick Sepsis-related Organ Failure Assessment (qSOFA) is a mortality predictor (Singer et al., 2016). Evidence of organ effects (and more serious sepsis) includes finding two of the three following criteria (Singer et al., 2016):

- Respiratory rate (RR) > 22 bpm
- Systolic blood pressure (SPB) < 100 mmHg
- Altered mental status

INTRAOSSEOUS ACCESS DEVICES

Intraosseous (IO) provides access to the noncollapsible venous plexus in the bone marrow space, thus enabling drug delivery similar to that achieved by central venous access. IO cannulation is now appropriate for settings when IV access cannot be obtained, and the patient would be compromised without the medication or solutions that have been prescribed for an emergent clinical condition (including rapid response team algorithms). There is limited information, but a case study and animal studies indicate that the IO site can be used for IV contrast dye in adults if there is no IV access available. Concerns still exist if a power injection should be used.

The Infusion Nurses Society (INS) Position Paper indicates a qualified registered nurse may insert, maintain, and remove IO access devices. The RN (depending on the state's Nurse Practice Act) must be:

- Proficient in infusion therapy
- Appropriately trained for the procedure (Phillips et al., 2010)

ALCOHOLISM/ALCOHOL WITHDRAWAL

Around 18 million people in the United States have an alcohol use disorder. Monitor admitted patients, especially those who had an unplanned admission (such as through the ED), for potential alcohol withdrawal. The onset for delirium tremors (DTs) is 6 to 8 hours after the last drink. Alcohol withdrawal seizures can occur 6 to 96 hours *after* the last drink. Use the Clinical Institute Withdrawal Assessment for Alcohol, Revised (CTWA-Ar). Items assessed include nausea/vomiting, tremor, paroxysmal sweats, tactile, auditory, or visual disturbances, anxiety, headache, agitation, and orientation. Consider the risk of alcohol-induced hypoglycemia (AIH) from insufficient glycogen stores and the alcohol-induced impairment of gluconeogenesis. It occurs during intoxication or up to 20 hours after the last drink (NIAAA, 2013).

Patients at risk for AIH are chronic alcoholics, binge drinkers, and young children.

LOCATION OF INTRAMUSCULAR INJECTIONS

- Intramuscular (IM) injections larger than 1 mL (for those aged 7 months or older) are given in the ventrogluteal area (gluteus medius, anterior gluteal site), not dorsogluteal (butt, upper outer quadrant, gluteus maximus).
- Even a properly located dorsogluteal injection still has the risk of nerve or artery injury.
- The ventrogluteal site has no major complications ever attributed to it because it avoids all major nerves and blood vessels.
- In addition, the body's fat is more evenly distributed, making it a shorter distance to reach the muscle.

Procedure to Locate Ventrogluteal

- Palpate the greater trochanter (feels like a golf ball).
- Place the palm of your hand on top of the trochanter.
- Position the index finger on or pointing toward the anterior superior iliac spine.
- Spread apart the third finger from the index finger.
- Administer the injection in the center of the "V" or triangle formed by the two fingers.

Hints for the Best IM Injection Technique

- Positioning the patient either in Sim's position (side-lying patient with top leg in front of bottom leg with knee bent) or prone with the toes pointed inward
- Applying manual pressure firmly for 10 seconds before inserting the needle (It stimulates the surrounding nerve endings.)
- Inserting the needle at a 90° insertion angle
- Stretching, rather than pinching, the skin (unless emaciated)
- Using Z-track technique (displacing the skin by 2.5–3.75 cm laterally before puncturing it, releasing and withdrawing the needle to "seal off" the site)
- Depressing the plunger slowly at a rate of 10 seconds per mL to allow the fluid to absorb

- Unless dorsogluteal is used, there is no need to aspirate for *any* injection

References

Bankhead, R., Boullata, J., Brantley, S., Corkins, M., Guenter, P., Krenitsky, J., & Wessel, J.; A.S.P.E.N. Board of Directors and the Enteral Nutrition Practice Recommendations Task Force. (2009). Enteral nutrition practice recommendations. *Journal of Parenteral Enteral Nutrition, 33*, 122–167. doi:10.1177/0148607108330314

Chen, L. L., & Lim, F. (2018). Routine supplemental oxygen for AMI: Modern-day myth. *Nursing, 48*(11), 19. doi:10.1097/01.NURSE.0000546472.87509.e4

Chung, F., Yegneswaran, B., Liao, P., Chung, S. A., Vairavanathan, S., Islam, S., & Shapiro, C. M. (2008). STOP questionnaire: A tool to screen patients for obstructive sleep apnea. *Anesthesiology, 108*(5), 812–821. doi:10.1097/ALN.0b013e31816d83e4

ENA 2015 Trauma Committee. (2016). *ENA topic brief: Avoiding the log roll maneuver: Alternative methods for safe patient handling.* Des Plaines, IL: Author.

Lester, D., Hartjes, T., & Bennett, A. (2018). A review of the revised sepsis care bundles. *American Journal of Nursing, 118*(8), 40–50. doi:10.1097/01.NAJ.0000544139.63510.b5

National Institute of Alcohol Abuse and Alcoholism. (2013). *Alcohol use disorder.* Retrieved from http://www.niaaa.nih.gov/alcohol-health/overview-alcohol-consumption/alcohol-use-disorders

Phillips, L., Brown, L., Campbell, T., Miller, J., Proehl, J., & Youngberg, B.; Consortium on Intraosseous Vascular Access in Healthcare Practice. (2010). Recommendations for the use of intraosseous vascular access for emergency and nonemergent situations in various healthcare settings: A consensus paper. *Journal of Emergency Nursing, 36*(6), 551–556. doi:10.1016/j.jen.2010.09.001

Siemieniuk, R. A. C., Chu, D. K., Kim, L. H., Güell-Rous, M. R., Alhazzani, W., Soccal, P. M., & Guyatt, G. H. (2018). Oxygen therapy for acutely ill medical patients: A clinical practice guideline. *BMJ, 363*, k4169. doi:10.1136/bmj.k4169

Singer, M., Deutshma, C. S., Seymour, C. W., Shanka-Hari, M., Annane, D., Bauer, M., & Angus, D. C. (2016). The third international census definitions for sepsis and septic shock (Sepsis-3). *JAMA, 315*(8), 801–810. doi:10.1001/jama.2016.0287

5

Safety and Civility in Radiology

Valerie Aarne Grossman

The radiology department is not immune to employees who lack positive, professional communication skills and attitudes. Without these skills at the center of all care provided, the risk to patient safety escalates. Research has shown that teams must work together in a professional manner to reach zero harm.

In this chapter, you will discover:

1. Effects of incivility on others
2. The financial, personal, and safety cost of incivility
3. Strategies to combat incivility

Radiology departments consist of many variables, from patient populations, different imaging technologies, job duties, licensure types to educational levels, while also being held to adhere to the rigorous standards of numerous governing agencies. This great mixture can easily lead to differing perspectives, objectives, and beliefs (Grossman, 2013). Organizations must stand firm and promote their mission and vision statements, assist their teams in meeting established expectations, and promote an environment of safety.

Leadership, teamwork, and personal accountability are essential to the success of every organization. Each team member is subjected to a variety of stressors. Depending on the individual, they will respond with either negative or positive behaviors (Bartholomew,

2006). Coping skills, mental health, and individual lifestyles additionally add complexities to each person's ability to maintain the highest standard of professionalism.

In 2009, The Joint Commission (TJC) established a Code of Conduct, setting forth principles and standards to guide employee behaviors. Leadership Standard LD 03.01.01 outlined the expectation that organizations should create a collaborative work environment that maintains a safety culture through heightened quality expectations. The Joint Commission stated that disruptive and inappropriate behaviors undermine the safety culture of an organization. It went on to require leadership to address adverse behaviors, promote reporting of situations, and create a disciplinary process for those who violate professional behavior standards (TJC, 2008). TJC affirmed unacceptable behaviors could lead to patient care errors, result in poor patient satisfaction, increase healthcare costs, and cause an increase in staff turnover. TJC updated this standard in 2012, and it remains in force today.

No work environment is immune to the risk of incivility. A 2019 study of radiography faculty in the United States revealed 60% of the respondents experienced some degree of incivility (Clark & Wagner, 2019). Another study involving medical imaging leaders and technologists concluded that conflict within radiology departments often led to avoidance of the situation or person, fear of physical harm from a coworker, and ultimately a delay in conflict resolution. Furthermore, these situations placed additional risk to patient safety, as coworkers who would not communicate professionally with each other failed to hand off important information regarding the patient to the next caretaker (Patton, 2018).

Many organizational factors contribute to the negative behavior of employees, leading to increased stress, decreased patience, ineffective coping skills, and, ultimately, inappropriate reactions to situations. These include:

- Increasing workload and productivity demands
- Cost-containment initiatives
- Fear of retaliation from leadership or coworkers
- Employee fatigue
- Lack of available resources to complete work appropriately
- Competing priorities
- Too many distractions
- Short staffing and/or high patient census
- Team culture that permits cruelty toward others
- Leadership failure to maintain high standards within the team
- Malfunction of essential equipment

Some negative behavior may be suggestive, well hidden from observers, or misinterpreted. A substantial amount of uncivil or bullying behavior is possible and could undermine a department's safety culture. These behaviors include:

- Nonverbal gestures (rolling eyes, facial expressions, raising eyebrows, slamming door, etc.)
- Failure to respect colleagues
  - Uncooperative attitudes
  - Betraying confidence
  - Blaming others instead of taking personal accountability
  - Forming of cliques or groups that exclude others
  - Retaliation toward the victim
  - Purposely setting a colleague up to fail
  - Slamming the phone on a caller or hanging up on someone
  - False allegations
  - Laughing at or teasing the victim
  - Rude or discourteous behavior or speech
  - Frequent criticism of environment, other people, organizational expectations, and so on
- Inappropriate methods of speaking
  - Verbal outburst or yelling at another person
  - Impatience with questions
  - Refusing to answer questions ("silent treatment")
  - Failure or refusal to return phone calls
  - Condescension or using vulgar language
  - Complaining about the target to others
  - Belittling, scapegoating, lying about the targeted person
  - Arguing
  - Rude comments
- Physical threats (real or implied)
- Sabotage of work being performed

Fast Facts

If negative behavior, incivility, and bullying are allowed in an organization, there will ultimately be a higher staff turnover rate, lower patient satisfaction scores, increase in serious safety events, and increased loss of revenue to the organization.

Individual characteristics that lead to negative behavior, incivility, or bullying toward others:

- Narcissism
- Immaturity
- Defensiveness
- Chemical dependency
- Mental illness
- History of being a victim (then becomes the perpetrator)
- Seeks to be in control of all activities (work-related, patient flow, social events, etc.)
- Lies easily and without remorse
- Inflated sense of self
- Sociopathic characteristics
    - Intelligent and well-spoken
    - Expert at manipulating others
    - Lacks empathy, shame, guilt, and so forth
    - Paranoia

A hostile work environment has negative effects on the targeted victim(s), including:

- Decreased self-esteem, withdrawal, or silence
- Defensiveness
- High rate of employee turnover
- Anxiety and/or depression
- Exhaustion
- Increased absenteeism
- Suicidal or homicidal ideation
- Physical illness (cardiac, gastrointestinal [GI] problems, migraine, etc.)
- Decrease in team commitment, picking up extra shifts, creativity, professional interest, and the like

Beliefs of the perpetrator ("bully"):

- If those around them are silent, they perceive their behavior is acceptable.
- If leadership fails to hold the perpetrator accountable, they believe their behavior is in line with the organizational expectations (Ciocco, 2018).

Effects upon the organization when incivility is permitted:

- Decreased productivity of employees
- Decreased quality of work performed
- High staff turnover
- Decreased customer satisfaction (employees take frustration out on patients)
- Risk of litigation

- High financial cost (In 2013, it was estimated that workplace incivility cost $24 billion annually in the United States.)
- Increased error rate as well as serious safety events (Gould, 2018; Hoffman & Chunta, 2015; Laschinger, Wong, Regan, Young-Ritchie, & Bushell, 2013; Porath & Pearson, 2013)

Fast Facts

If uncivil behavior is allowed to continue, the perpetrator believes their behavior is in line with the organizational mission and vision.

To build a culture promoting safety and professionalism, organizations must enforce zero-tolerance of unacceptable behaviors. From established policies to ongoing, formal in-servicing, organizational leadership must address issues that can, at times, be difficult and uncomfortable.

Policies
- Should include a "nonretaliation" clause
- Thorough investigation of all reports of incivility
- Avoid double standards (All employees must be held to the same standard regardless of their profitability, protected status, kinship, role within the organization, etc.)

Education
- Skill-based coaching for all leaders
- Ongoing in-servicing for all employees
- Cognitive rehearsal strategy, especially for less tenured staff

Safe Reporting
- Establish method for reporting unprofessional/unsafe situations
- Reduce fear of intimidation, retribution, and retaliation
- Allow anonymous reporting

Promote Accountability
- Offenders must be held accountable

Fast Facts

Cognitive rehearsal is a strategy for targeted individuals to implement when being attacked by another individual (Longo, 2017). This is a learned strategy that is practiced in advance, with a predetermined response that is used when being a target of incivility.

References

Bartholomew, K. (2006). *Ending nurse-to-nurse hostility*. Marblehead, MA: HCPro, Inc..

Ciocco, M. (2018). *Fast facts on combating nurse bullying, incivility, and workplace violence*. New York, NY: Springer Publishing Company.

Clark, K., & Wagner, J. (2019). Incivility among radiography educators in the United States. *The Internet Journal of Allied Health Sciences and Practice, 17*(3), Article 2.

Gould, T. (2018). Workplace bullies: Watch out for these 8 personality types. *HR Morning*. Retrieved from https://www.hrmorning.com/articles/8-workplace-bully-personality-types/

Grossman, V. A. (2013). Hot topics: Teamwork essentials: Success in the radiology environment. *Journal of Radiology Nursing, 32*, 139–140. doi:10.1016/j.jradnu.2013.03.002

Hoffman, R., & Chunta, K. (2015). Workplace incivility: Promoting zero tolerance in nursing. *Journal of Radiology Nursing, 34*(4), 222–227. doi:10.1016/j.jradnu.2015.09.004

Laschinger, H., Wong, C., Regan, S., Young-Ritchie, C., & Bushell, P. (2013). Workplace incivility and new graduate nurse's mental health: The protective role of resiliency. *Journal of Nursing Administration, 43*(7–8), 415–421. doi:10.1097/NNA.0b013e31829d61c6

Longo, J. (2017, August 30). Cognitive rehearsal: Learn a strategy for addressing incivility and bulling in nursing. *American Nurse Today*. Retrieved from https://www.americannursetoday.com/cognitive-rehearsal/

Patton, C. (2018). Workplace conflict: It matters how staff deal with it. *Health Management, 18*(5), 352–354. Retrieved from https://healthmanagement.org/c/healthmanagement/issuearticle/workplace-conflict

Porath, C., & Pearson, C. (2013, January–February). Motivating people: The price of incivility. *The Harvard Business Review*. Retrieved from https://hbr.org/2013/01/the-price-of-incivility

The Joint Commission. (2008, July 9). Behaviors that undermine a culture of safety. *Sentinel Event Alert* (40). Retrieved from https://www.jointcommission.org/sentinel_event_alert_issue_40_behaviors_that_undermine_a_culture_of_safety/

II

Nursing Essentials

6

Vascular Access Device Care and Management

Jong Hee Oh

When preparing a patient for an imaging or procedural visit to a radiology department, the nurse must be skilled in assessing the vascular access needs of the patient. Precision skills and expertise are essential in providing the highest quality and safest care to the patient.

In this chapter, you will discover:

- Peripheral intravenous catheters (PIV)
- Midline catheters and central venous catheters (CVC)
- Intraosseous catheters

VASCULAR ACCESS DEVICE CARE AND MANAGEMENT

Radiology departments have various customers to consider in providing imaging services and therapeutic procedures. Customers may visit radiology for an imaging test or procedure from a different point of care, such as home, the physician's office, a skilled nursing facility, the hospital, or an ED. In this clinical setting, the majority of customers are required to have a vascular access device to have their tests or procedures performed. To serve these customers effectively, the radiology nurse needs to be equipped with the most up-to-date knowledge and skills to manage the various types of vascular access devices.

The essential role of the radiology nurse is to prepare customers based on their radiologic needs. This includes understanding imaging tests and procedures, identifying the necessity of venous access, assessing patients' vasculature, and providing appropriate venous access and care. Nurses must understand how the combination of radiographic technology and a venous access device can either help accurately diagnose medical conditions or result in potential complications such as infiltration or extravasation. To provide quality care and prevent potential complications from occurring, nurses must utilize evidence-based practice.

Fast Facts

When utilizing a patient's vascular access for a radiologic purpose, be familiar with the institutional guidelines, the manufacturer's recommendations of that product (e.g., PIVs, midline catheters, CVCs, intraosseous catheters, power injection, contrast essentials), governing entities (organizational policies, State Nurse Practice Act, U.S. Food and Drug Administration regulations, The Joint Commission), as well as professional organizations (e.g., Infusion Nurses Society [INS], Association of periOperative Registered Nurses [AORN], Association for Radiologic & Imaging Nursing [ARIN], and American College of Radiology [ACR]).

Vascular Access Device Options

- PIV
- Midline catheters: a vascular access device measuring 8 inches or less with the distal tip located at or below the level of axilla
- CVCs: peripherally inserted central catheters (PICC), nontunneled CVCs, tunneled CVCs, implanted ports

Peripheral Intravenous Catheters

- Discuss with a patient about arm preference for PIV site selection.
- Determine any contraindications for a PIV insertion, such as breast surgery with axillary node dissection, lymphedema, an arteriovenous fistula graft, an affected extremity from a cerebrovascular accident, or chronic kidney disease (Infusion Nurse Society, 2016).

- Identify the most appropriate size of the catheter needed to safely perform the study:
  - Common sizes for use in adults are 22 gauge, 20 gauge, and 18 gauge.
  - In adults, a 20-gauge power rated catheter in antecubital fossa or forearm is preferable for CT power injection (flow rates of 3 mL/sec or higher).
  - A 22-gauge power rated catheter can be used for the CT injection, adjusting the flow rate to <3.0 mL/sec in adults and <2.0 mL/sec in pediatric patients (American College of Radiology, 2018).
- Verify placement and optimal functioning of the catheter prior to use.
  - When inserting PIV, ensure its placement by checking blood flashback and PIV insertion site by flushing the catheter with a normal saline flush.
  - For an existing IV, brisk blood return from catheter can be the main indicator of its functionality.
- Vein selections for power injection:
  - The optimal PIV site is an antecubital fossa or large forearm vein (ACR, 2018).
  - Avoid PIVs placed in areas of flexion, feet, hands, or external jugular (INS, 2016).
- Special considerations for PIV insertions:
  - Use vascular visualization technology such as near infrared and ultrasound for patients with difficult venous access (INS, 2016).
  - Utilize some of the commonly used techniques for patients with limited venous access.
    - Use gravity to help the venous filling.
    - Use heat pack for 10 to 15 minutes to dilates the vein.
    - Use a blood pressure cuff to distribute pressure evenly and to distend the vein; limit pressure below a diastolic pressure of less than 80 mmHg and maintain arterial circulation (INS, 2016).
- Identify the patient using two patient identifiers to avoid unnecessary procedure or patient harm.
- Gather supplies needed.
- Use appropriate hand hygiene by washing hands with soap and water or with alcohol-based hand rubs.
- Use disposable clean gloves.
- Prepare skin with an antiseptic before PIV insertion; chlorhexidine in alcohol solution is preferable as a skin prep agent. Tincture of iodine, iodophor (povidone-iodine), or 70% alcohol prep may also be used (Centers for Disease Control and Prevention, 2011).

- Use a "no-touch" technique for PIV insertion after applying skin prep to maintain sterility of insertion site (INS, 2016).

Midline Catheters and CVCs

- Follow institutional practice guidelines and manufacturers' recommendations for safe use.
- For the CT exam, determine if the midline or CVC is compatible with IV contrast media and is power rated.
- Special considerations for midline catheters and CVCs:
    - Identify the patient using two patient identifiers.
    - Use appropriate hand hygiene.
    - Confirm CVC tip location before injecting IV contrast media. The optimal tip location is the lower one-third of the superior vena cava or cavoatrial junction.
    - Verify patency of catheter by checking brisk blood return with a 10 mL normal saline flush.
    - Flush a lumen of catheter with preservative-free 0.9% normal saline solution before and after injecting IV contrast media.
    - Use aseptic technique when accessing a lumen of CVC and follow infection-prevention steps (INS, 2016).

Intraosseous Catheters

- Increasing in popularity among emergency response teams (inside of hospitals as well as prehospital care).

Recent case studies indicate that contrast medium can be safely injected using intraosseous access (Ahrens, Reeder, Keevil, & Tupesis, 2013; Budach & Niehues, 2017).

References

Ahrens, K. L., Reeder, S. B., Keevil, J. G., & Tupesis, J. P. (2013). Successful computed tomography angiogram through tibial intraosseous access: A case report. *The Journal of Emergency Medicine, 45*(2), 182–185. doi:10/1016/j.jemermed.2012.11.091

American College of Radiology. (2018). *ACR manual on contrast. Version 10.3*. Retrieved from https://www.acr.org/-/media/ACR/Files/Clinical-Resources/Contrast_Media.pdf

Budach, N. M., & Niehues, S. M. (2017). CT angiography of the chest and abdomen in an emergency patient via humeral intraosseous access. *Emergency Radiology, 24*(1), 105–108. doi:10.1007/s10140-016-1438-6

Centers for Disease Control and Prevention. (2011). *Guidelines for the prevention of intravascular catheter-related infections*. Retrieved from https://www.cdc.gov/hicpac/pdf/guidelines/bsi-guidelines-2011.pdf

Infusion Nurse Society. (2016). Infusion therapy standards of practice. *Journal of Infusion Nursing, 39*(1), S54.

7

Sedation and Monitoring

Lora K. (Ott) Hromadik

Procedural sedation and patient monitoring are central to the role of the radiology nurse. Safe patient care in radiology requires radiology nurses to be knowledgeable in the care of the patient from the intrahospital transport of acutely ill patients to radiology and the care of the patient from presedation through postsedation patient monitoring and medication administration. Additionally, the radiology nurse provides important interventions when adverse events occur and patients are at risk of harm.

In this chapter, you will discover:

1. Types of monitoring equipment and purposes
2. Types of procedural sedation and analgesia (PSA)
3. Recovery process and interventions

Guidelines for the intrahospital transport of ICU patients have been established by the Society of Critical Care Medicine and the American College of Critical Care Medicine (Table 7.1). The guidelines require five levels of consideration for maintaining ICU level care and monitoring of critically ill patients while in the radiology department.

Patients requiring cardiac monitoring in the acute care setting (non-ICU) require cardiac monitoring during hospital transport and in the radiology setting. The discontinuation of monitoring for transport and radiological care requires a physician order or a preestablished protocol to establish safe off-monitor transport (Ott, 2015).

Fast Facts

There are no national guidelines established for the transport of non-critically ill acute care patients (non-ICU). However, the ICU guidelines can be applied to non-ICU patients.

Table 7.1

Intrahospital Transport of ICU Patient Guidelines

Patient Needs	Nursing Actions
Preplanning	Coordination and communication with the ICU staff ■ Decrease any waiting time in the radiology department ■ Decrease disruption to the patient treatments Establish appropriateness of the procedure ■ The need for contrast ■ The need for the exam outweighs the risk of transport out of the ICU Scheduling appropriate personnel ■ Respiratory therapist ■ ICU-level RN ■ Critical care medicine physician, if needed Establish procedural risks ■ MRI screening ■ Life-supporting intravenous drips ■ Ability of patient to lie flat, remain still, hold their breath Contrast dye allergies ■ Scheduling contrast premedication ■ Appropriate IV access
Personnel	Minimum of two people trained in intrahospital transport ■ Minimum of one certified in resuscitation ■ ICU-trained RN ■ Respiratory therapy for all ventilated patients ■ Physician for all unstable patients
Equipment	Equipment to maintain ICU level of care ■ Transport monitors, including invasive monitors ■ Ventilators and airway management ■ Drug infusions with properly maintained equipment ■ Identify the location of crash carts en route to the radiology department

(continued)

Table 7.1

Intrahospital Transport of ICU Patient Guidelines (*continued*)	
Patient Needs	**Nursing Actions**
Monitoring	Maintain the same level of physiologic monitoring as was being received in the ICU
	▪ Blood pressure
	▪ Pulse oximetry
	▪ Cardiac monitoring
	▪ Arterial lines
Documentation	Maintain a record of patient data
	▪ Vital signs
	▪ Procedures
	▪ Medications
	▪ Patient response

Source: Data from Warren, J., Fromm, R., Orr, R., Rotello, L., Horst, M., & American College of Critical Care Medicine. (2004). Guidelines for the inter- and intrahospital transport of critically ill patients. *Critical Care Medicine, 32*(1), 256–262. doi:10.1097/01. CCM.0000104917.39204.0A

PROCEDURAL SEDATION AND ANALGESIA

Goals/Purposes

PSA provides a means for patients to tolerate painful procedures or procedures requiring them not to move without undergoing the risks of general anesthesia. Patients undergoing procedural sedation should be able to respond to verbal commands and tactile stimulation. Sedation can be categorized into four levels. The goals for PSA are to provide an altered level of consciousness or anxiety, to elevate the pain threshold with possible amnesia of unpleasant events while maintaining a protected airway, to ensure stable blood pressure and heart rate, and to return the patient to presedation state prior to discharge. The radiology nurse is responsible for administering minimal and moderate sedation to achieve these goals (Table 7.2).

Preparation for PSA

Safe administration of PSA requires proper preparation before any medications are administered (see Table 7.3).

Table 7.2

Levels of Sedation

Level of Sedation	Response to Verbal and Tactile Stimuli	Maintains Airway	Spontaneous Ventilation	Maintains Heart Rate and Blood Pressure
Minimal (anxiolysis)	Normal	Yes	Yes	Yes
Moderate (conscious)	Purposeful	Yes	Yes	Usually
Deep	Repeated verbal and/or painful stimuli required	May require intervention	May be inadequate	Usually
General anesthesia	Unresponsive to painful stimuli	Often requires intervention	Often inadequate	May be impaired

Source: Adapted from Meyers, J. L., & Chaudhuri, S. (2011). Procedural sedation and analgesia: A practical review for non-anesthesiologists. *Journal of Surgical Radiology,* 2(4), 344–356.

Table 7.3

Preparation for Procedural Sedation and Analgesia

Patient Preparation for Procedural Sedation and Analgesia

Action	Details
Consent	Informed consent obtained by the physician after being informed of the risks, benefits, limitations, and possible alternatives to procedural sedation.
NPO	Fasting guidelines allow for adequate gastric emptying, 2 hours for clear liquids, 6 hours for a light meal, 8 hours for a regular meal.
Intravenous access	Intravenous access should be maintained throughout the procedure and until the patient is no longer at risk for cardiovascular or respiratory depression.
Supplemental oxygen	Oxygenation via nasal cannula or an alternative appropriate delivery system to decrease the risk of hypoxia during moderate sedation. Recommended by the ASA for all patients receiving moderate sedation.

(continued)

Table 7.3

Preparation for Procedural Sedation and Analgesia (*continued*)	
Emergency equipment/room preparation	Monitoring equipment, suctioning, and oxygen delivery equipment are present and in good working order. Resuscitation drugs and fluids, defibrillator, intubation supplies, Ambu bag, and mask readily available.
Personnel	One ACLS-trained person is designated responsible for sedation.

ACLS, advanced cardiac life support; ASA, American Society of Anesthesiologists.
Source: Adapted from Meyers, J. L., & Chaudhuri, S. (2011). Procedural sedation and analgesia: A practical review for non-anesthesiologists. *Journal of Surgical Radiology,* 2(4), 344–356.

Preprocedural Evaluation by the Physician

- A current history and physical including past medical history, review of the systems, allergies, medications, and an airway assessment should be done by a physician.
- Documentation of use of marijuana for medical or recreational use and any illicit drug use.
- The physical examination and vital signs should be updated just prior to the sedation.
- A physician should assign an American Society of Anesthesiologists (ASA) score based on the patient's general health (see Table 7.4).

Table 7.4

American Society of Anesthesiologists Score		
ASA Level	**Description**	**Risk**
1	Healthy patient	Low
2	Mild systemic disease	Low
3	Severe systemic disease	High
4	Severe systemic disease that threatens life	High
5	Dying patient not expected to survive without procedure	High
6	Brain-dead patient for organ harvesting for donation	
E	Designates the procedure as an emergency	High

ASA, American Society of Anesthesiologists.

MONITORING AND SEDATION MEDICATIONS

- In addition to respiratory suppression, the medications used for PSA may suppress the autonomic nervous system's ability to adequately respond to hypovolemia; therefore, close monitoring of vital signs is important for the safe well-being of patients (Kaye, Kaye, & Urman, 2015). Refer to Table 7.5 for the recommended monitoring type and intervals.
- Continuous electrocardiographic monitoring (EKG) and 1:1 nursing surveillance are indicated with moderate sedation (Landrum, 2014).
- The most common anxiolytic medications used during procedures are benzodiazepines.
  - Midazolam for moderate sedation and diazepam or lorazepam for mild sedation. (For information on EKG interpretation, *Fast Facts About EKGs for Nurses* [2014] by Michele Landrum, New York, NY: Springer Publishing Company.)
  - Flumazenil reliably reverses the amnesia, sedation, and respiratory depression caused by benzodiazepines and should be available whenever benzodiazepines are used for procedural sedation.

- The common analgesic medications used during procedures are opioids.
  - Fentanyl for moderate sedation and hydromorphone or morphine for mild sedation.
  - Naloxone reliably reverses the central nervous system depression caused by opioids and should be available whenever opioids are used for procedural sedation.

- Special consideration needs to be given to known marijuana (both medical and recreational) use and illicit drug use.
  - Marijuana depresses the autonomic nervous system response, thus perpetuating the physiologic response to PSA (Huson, Granados, & Rasko, 2018).
  - Marijuana is a fat-soluble drug known to continue a slow release into the body for as much as 30 days (Twardowski, Link, & Twardowski, 2019).
  - Chronic opioid use decreases the effectiveness of opioids used in PSA; thus, higher doses may be needed for effective sedation.

Fast Facts

- An informed patient is more cooperative and needs less sedation.
- Sedation cannot make up for poor technique.

(continued)

(*continued*)

- "Less is more": It is easier and safer to add smaller doses than to reverse what has already been given.
- Marijuana and chronic opioid use may affect the response to sedation medications.

Table 7.5

Monitoring Types and Intervals

Monitored Vital Sign	Method	Frequency	Rationale
Level of consciousness	Provide verbal or tactile stimuli	Prior to administration of repeated doses of medications	Best indicator of sedation effect, best indicator of patient's ability to protect airway
Oxygenation	Pulse oximetry	Continuous	Early identification of hypoxia
Ventilation	Respiratory rate, capnography for moderate and deep sedation	Every 5 minutes, continuous with capnography	Direct observation of frequency and quality of respiratory effort
Circulation	Heart rate, blood pressure, and EKG monitoring	Every 5 minutes, heart rate and blood pressure, EKG continuous	Early recognition of hypovolemia
Temperature	Oral and skin temperature	Once prior to, during, and after procedure	Identification of temperature fluctuations
Level of Sedation	0—None 1—Minimal 2—Moderate 3—Deep sedation 4—General anesthesia	Every 5 minutes	To prevent oversedation and early identification of the need for emergency intervention

POSTRECOVERY CARE AND DISCHARGE

PSA medications promote a rapid recovery stage with minimal postprocedure impairment. The recovery and discharge process will be institution specific. Patients need to be observed until there is no risk of cardio-respiratory depression or compromise. Monitor vital signs, including level of consciousness, and, if needed, intervene quickly with resuscitation efforts. An ACLS-trained nurse needs to attend to the recovery process until the patient is stable, meeting the discharge criteria set by the individual institution. Examples of discharge criteria are the Aldrete Scoring System and the postanesthesia discharge scoring system. See Table 7.6.

Table 7.6

Postprocedure Recovery Score

Postanesthesia Discharge Scoring System		Aldrete Scoring System	
Vital signs		Activity: able to move, voluntarily or on command	
Within 20% of preoperative values	2	Four extremities	2
20–40%	1	Two extremities	1
40%	0	No extremities	0
Activity/mental status		Respiration	
Oriented and steady gait	2	Able to breathe deeply and cough freely	2
Oriented or steady gait	1	Dyspnea, swallow, or irritated breathing	1
Neither	0	Apneic	0
Pain, nausea, emesis		Circulation	
Minimal	2	BP +/- 20 mmHg of pre-PSA level	2
Moderate	1	BP +/- 20 – 49 mmHg of pre-PSA level	1
Severe	0	BP + 50 mmHg of preoperative level	0
Bleeding		Consciousness	
Minimal	2	Fully awake	2
Moderate	1	Arousable on calling	1
Severe	0	Unresponsive	0
Intake and output		Oxygen saturation	
PO fluids and voided	2	Normal, pink	2
PO fluids or voided	1	Pale, dusky, blotchy	1
Neither	0	Cyanotic	0
Score ≥ 9 needed for safe discharge to home		Score ≥ 9 points required for recovery confirmed	

Source: Data from Meyers, J. L., & Chaudhuri, S. (2011). Procedural sedation and analgesia: A practical review for non-anesthesiologists. *Journal of Surgical Radiology, 2*(4), 344–356.

Prior to discharge, the patients should

- be alert, oriented, and at baseline;
- be discharged with a responsible adult who will be the designated driver, assume the care for the patient, and recognize and communicate complications;
- be provided with written discharge instructions, follow-up care, and emergency contact numbers; and
- retain a signed copy of the discharge instructions for the medical record.

RAPID RESPONSE SYSTEM

The rapid response system (RRS) provides critical care expertise when ICU level care is needed for compromised patients outside of the ICU, including radiology. The RRS is a radiology nurse's resource when patients have adverse reactions to sedation, procedures, or diagnostic tests. Studies by Ott et al. (2012) and Tindal, Darby, and Simmons (2014) conducted in radiology have shown that the most common causes of patient deterioration requiring RRS intervention were

- cardiac (such as hypotension, tachycardia, chest pain);
- respiratory (such as hypoxia, dyspnea, pulmonary edema); and
- neurologic (such as altered level of consciousness, stroke, seizure) in nature.

The radiology nurse becomes a member of the RRS once the system intervenes on the patient's behalf (see Box 7.1).

Box 7.1 Radiology Nurses' Responsibility to the Rapid Response System (RRS)

- Know the institution's RRS call criteria—post and make visible to all staff.
- Continual surveillance of sedated patients facilitates rapid RRS deployment.
- Nonsedated radiology patients are also at risk for requiring the RRS; identify patients at greatest risk for compromise for rapid RRS deployment should call criteria be met.
- Participate with the RRS by providing history of care and events prior to the RRS call.
- Record and document RRS call, treatments, and outcomes.
- Keep the patient and family informed of what is taking place and why.

Fast Facts

Call the RRS when patients meet call criteria. *Delay jeopardizes patient safety.*

References

Huson, H., Granados, T., & Rasko, Y. (2018). Surgical considerations of marijuana use in elective procedures. *Heliyon, 4*(9), e00779. doi:10.1016/j.heliyon.2018.e00779

Kaye, A. D., Kaye, A. M., & Urman, R. D. (Eds.). (2015). *Essentials of pharmacology for anesthesia, pain medicine, and critical care.* New York, NY: Springer Publishing Company.

Landrum, M. (2014). *Fast facts about EKGs for nurses.* New York, NY: Springer Publishing Company.

Meyers, J. L., & Chaudhuri, S. (2011). Procedural sedation and analgesia: A practical review for non-anesthesiologists. *Journal of Surgical Radiology, 2*(4), 344–356.

Ott, L. (2015). Shielding from harm: When is it ok to send a patient to radiology off monitor? *Journal of Radiology Nursing, 34*(4), 242–244. doi:10.1016/j.jradnu.2015.10.002

Ott, L., Pinsky, M., Hoffman, L., Clarke, S., Clark, S., Ren, D., & Hravnak, M. (2012). Medical emergency team calls in the radiology department: Patient characteristics and outcomes. *BMJ Quality and Safety, 21*(6), 509–518. doi:10.1136/bmjqs-2011-000423

Tindal, M., Darby, J., & Simmons, R. (2014). A retrospective review of crisis events in diagnostic radiology: An analysis of frequency, demographics, etiologies, and outcomes. *Journal of Patient Safety, 10*(2), 111–116. doi:10.1097/PTS.0000000000000113

Twardowski, M., Link, M., & Twardowski, N. (2019). Effects of cannabis use on sedation requirements for endoscopic procedures. *The Journal of the American Osteopathic Association, 119*(5), 307–311. doi:10.7556/jaoa.2019.052

Warren, J., Fromm, R., Orr, R., Rotello, L., Horst, M., & American College of Critical Care Medicine. (2004). Guidelines for the inter- and intra-hospital transport of critically ill patients. *Critical Care Medicine, 32*(1), 256–262. doi:10.1097/01.CCM.0000104917.39204.0A

8

Documentation

Brooke Grandusky

In the nursing profession, there is an old saying: "If you didn't document it, then it wasn't done." Nurses working in a fast-paced radiology environment must have the skills to document clearly and concisely the timeline of care delivered and the patient's response to the care. The radiology nurse's documentation is essential to capture the "story" of the interventional radiology (IR) procedure or assist the provider in what to include in the dictation of the exam report. The radiology nurse needs to document timely assessments and assume the care of the patient while away from the ED, inpatient unit, or in a procedural/imaging area.

In this chapter, you will discover:

1. Purpose of electronic medical records (EMRs)
2. Integration of patient care with electronic documentation
3. Terminology associated with electronic documentation

Because of federal legislation and regulatory requirements, most documentation done in patient care settings is now electronic. EMRs are designed so that documentation is easier, focused, inclusive, and more standardized. EMR documentation also provides valuable tools for reporting data and improving care. Clinicians can access patient data across a variety of care settings such as the ED, inpatient, and ambulatory care settings. As EMR vendors make improvements, there is the ability to have a completely integrated chart as well as the functionality to view care given at another facility.

EMR documentation has opened up many opportunities to improve documentation and communication between the radiology department and primary care teams. Hand-off reports can be documented electronically, and radiology nurses can document on the same medication administration record (MAR) used in inpatient and ambulatory settings. The EMR supports both the inpatient and ambulatory care providers in accessing image links and both the preliminary and final reports.

Fast Facts

Forthcoming changes in the healthcare world stress the importance of accurate and complete documentation. Payment for high-tech diagnostic exams will depend on the documentation supporting the necessity of the exam. While the bedside RN may not see the implications of omitting information or rushing through a health history, the patient may feel the impact when they get a bill for services denied. The documented information not only helps guide the care of the patient, it also justifies the necessity of the care.

If the picture archiving and communication system (PACS) and the radiology information system (RIS) are separate, there must be thoughtful decisions on how to best document the care of the patient while in radiology. Departmental workflows and customized documentation tools are very important. Integration of the various computer systems with the EMR being used is imperative.

Clinical staff should be deeply involved in building the EMR and deciding how the EMR should be used at the bedside. The diverse modalities in radiology may add EMR documentation challenges for the nurse. For example, the nurse in CT documents differently from the nurse in MRI. The IR nurse administers moderate sedation, while monitoring the patient and the nurse in nuclear medicine may need to assist by the injecting of radiopharmaceuticals into a central venous catheter. All actions are different, and the radiology nurse will need the ability to use an EMR system that will allow appropriate documentation of nursing care delivered. EMRs also make it "easier" to audit a chart, but with so much information now available and so many ways to document the same thing, clinicians need to establish documentation standards and workflows.

Much of the documentation in a radiology setting may be captured in an electronic format, while some departments may still use paper for some actions.

RADIOLOGY EMR DOCUMENTATION TERMS

- Radiology information system (RIS)
  - Information systems, usually computer assisted, designed to store, manipulate, and retrieve information for planning, organizing, directing, and controlling administrative activities associated with the provision and utilization of radiology services and facilities (MedConditions, 2013).
- Picture archiving and communication system (PACS)
  - Imaging technology used to store and access images from multiple modalities.
  - Replaces film with electronically stored and displayed digital images.
- Electronic medical record (EMR)
  - Digital version of a paper chart that contains all of a patient's medical history from one practice.
  - Mostly used by providers for diagnosis and treatment (healthit.gov).
- Electronic health records (EHRs)
  - Include a more comprehensive patient history and are designed to contain and share information from all providers involved in a patient's care.
  - Allow patient health to move with them (healthit.gov).
- Meaningful use (MU)
  - Set of standards defined by the Centers for Medicare and Medicaid Services (CMS) Incentive Programs that governs the use of EMRs and allows eligible providers/hospitals to earn incentive payments by meeting specific criteria (healthit.gov).
  - Goal of MU is to promote the use of EHRs and improve healthcare.
- Health Insurance Portability and Accountability Act of 1996 (HIPAA)
  - Protects the privacy of the patient's health information, regulates the security of electronic protected health information, mandates notification following a breach of unsecured protected health information, and ensures the protection of identifiable information, which may be used to analyze patient safety events and improve patient safety.

- Best Practice Advisory (BPA)
  - Communicated updates regarding a method or technique that has consistently shown results superior to those achieved with other means.
- Health Information Technology for Economic and Clinical Health (HITECH) Act:
  - The HITECH Act, enacted as part of the American Recovery and Reinvestment Act of 2009, was signed into law on February 17, 2009, to promote the adoption and meaningful use of health information technology.
  - Subtitle D of the HITECH Act addresses the privacy and security concerns associated with the electronic transmission of health information, in part, through several provisions that strengthen the civil and criminal enforcement of the HIPAA rules (http://www.hhs.gov/ocr/privacy/hipaa/administrative/enforcementrule/hitechenforcementifr.html).
- ARRA: The American Recovery and Reinvestment Act of 2009
- HIMSS: Healthcare Information and Management Systems Society
- ICD-10-CM/PCS: International Classification of Diseases, 10th Edition, Clinical Modification/Procedure Coding System. ICD-10 diagnosis codes are used to report medical diagnoses and inpatient procedures and were created by the World Health Organization. The deadline to transition into ICD-10 was October 1, 2014 (cms.gov).
- CMS: Centers for Medicare and Medicaid Services. Agency within the U.S. Department of Health and Human Services that oversees many key federal healthcare programs, including EHR incentive programs, MU, HIPAA, Medicare, and Medicaid.
- Successful documentation in radiology depends on several components, including:
  - Support of senior leadership
  - Attention to detail and impact of documentation upon workflows
  - Adequate resources to document appropriately (time, equipment)
  - Documentation standards in place to guide staff.
  - MIPS: Merit-Based Incentive Payment System
  - PAMA: Protecting Access to Medicare Act

Fast Facts

The EMR is a *tool* to document care delivered. Staff need 24-7 access to technical support and enough computers available to document patient care. Although documentation in healthcare is essential, no tool should ever distract a staff member from the purpose of their work. Never lose sight that the "patient" in front of you is a human being who deserves your utmost compassion and attention.

Reference

MedConditions. (2013). *Dictionary of medical conditions terminology.* Retrieved from http://medconditions.net/

9

Legal Considerations in Radiology Nursing

Edith Brous

Radiology nursing requires particular skills and experience. In addition to the documentation and interpersonal skills that all nurses require, the radiology nurse must have the assessment and monitoring skills of a critical care nurse, the triage and rapid decision-making skills of an ED nurse, and the sterile technique and positioning skills of an operating nurse. Deficiencies in any of these areas can expose the radiology nurse to malpractice allegations as well as professional misconduct investigations.

In this chapter, you will discover:

1. The elements of a malpractice case
2. The purpose of nursing regulation
3. Tips to reduce liability exposure

MALPRACTICE

Persons alleging professional negligence against a radiology nurse must show that the nurse departed from acceptable standards of practice and that the departure caused harm to the patient. To prevail, a person bringing a lawsuit must demonstrate four required elements:

1. The radiology nurse had a *duty* to the patient.
2. The radiology nurse *breached* that duty.
3. The radiology nurse's breach of duty *caused* the patient's injury.
4. The patient suffered actual *harm*.

Liability exposure occurs when nurses bypass procedural safeguards, engage in "workarounds" in violation of organizational policies, or fail to accurately and adequately document their observations and communications. Some events in the radiology suite that can lead to allegations of professional malpractice include medication errors, falls, nerve damage from faulty positioning, iatrogenic infections, failure to monitor for, recognize, or respond to complications, foreign body retention, failure to protect patients from harm, or improper drain management.

Malpractice defense lawyers depend heavily upon the medical record. Entries that reflect adherence to organizational policies and the current standards of practice are essential in defending accused nurses. Communications between the nurse and the patient should document the patient's level of consciousness at the time of the conversation, any witnesses to the conversation, and the patient's ability to repeat given instructions. Entries regarding adverse events must indicate that the radiology nurse engaged the chain of command and pursued clinical concerns to resolution. Charting should be performed in a manner that allows the nurse to recreate an accurate sequence of events and a clinical picture of the patient by reading his or her entries in the future.

Fast Facts

Radiology nurses should always maintain a professional liability insurance policy and not solely rely on employer coverage.

LICENSURE

The mission of licensing boards is to protect the public from unsafe, impaired, incompetent, or unethical providers. Nursing regulation takes place at the state level to protect patients from nurses who can harm them. The board of nursing might be required by law to investigate every complaint made about a nurse. The board will close the case after an investigation if it finds no professional misconduct. If it does, discipline is likely to be imposed on the nurse's license. Such discipline can range from a private reprimand to revocation of the license. Licensure discipline also causes multiple collateral legal and professional problems. Nurses under investigation by their licensing boards should be represented by counsel at all stages of the investigation. For this reason, employer policies are not adequate to cover liability issues for nurses. Employer policies only provide coverage for lawsuits related to events arising in the course of the nurse's employment. This leaves the nurse uninsured for licensure discipline proceedings.

Some potential licensure discipline issues for radiology nurses include boundary violations, unsafe practice, substance use disorders or impaired practice, falsified documentation (including precharting), exceeding the scope of practice, failure to wear an identification badge indicating status, improper delegation, or any of the clinical performance issues that lead to malpractice lawsuits. Because scopes of practice differ in individual jurisdictions, radiology nurses must be familiar with the Nurse Practice Act in the state(s) in which they practice. Most such statutes are available on the nursing board's websites, and nurses should visit those sites periodically.

Fast Facts

With the exception of Michigan, nurses in all states and territories can look up, verify, and monitor any of their nursing licenses through the E-Notify notification system of Nursys® at Nursys.com.

INFORMED CONSENT

Although radiology nurses might be obligated to witness the patient's signature on a consent form or confirm consent forms are in the record prior to sedation or procedures, the responsibility to explain risks, benefits, alternatives, and costs of a procedure generally belongs to the person performing the procedure and exceeds the RN scope of practice. Nurses are responsible for educating patients and addressing their concerns. Radiology nurses also must document these conversations and show they have communicated patient concerns to anesthesia and the physician performing the procedure.

REDUCING LIABILITY EXPOSURE

Radiology nurses can reduce the potential for being named in a lawsuit or investigated by their nursing boards by incorporating the following into their usual and customary practice:

1. Revise clinical performance based upon practice standard and organizational policy changes.
2. Document in a manner that allows for future reconstruction of patient presentations and accurate chronology of events.
3. Hone interpersonal skills—patients are less likely to sue providers with whom they have a good relationship.
4. Study the Nurse Practice Act and definitions of professional misconduct in any state in which a license has ever been held. Nurses can still have reporting obligations in states in which their registration certificates are not current.
5. Identify unsafe conditions in writing.
6. Maintain cultural competency.

Fast Facts

Radiology nurses must exhibit continued competency and adherence to evidence-based standards of practice. Belonging to professional organizations and subscribing to professional journals can demonstrate commitment to this goal.

III

Radiologic Imaging Modalities: CT and MRI

10

Computed Axial Tomography Basics

Velecia Marston

A CT scan uses a combination of computer-processed images and measurements taken from different angles to produce cross-sectional images. This technology allows for the visualization of specific body areas without having to perform surgery.

In this chapter, you will discover:

1. Basic information regarding the CT scanner
2. Patient preparation for a CT scan
3. Essential patient education

CT SCANS

Computed axial tomography (CAT scan or CT scan) is a relatively "young" modality, first discussed in the 1970s. CT scans use computer-processed x-rays to create slices (aka tomographic images) of a specific body part. The early CT scanners took up to 20 minutes per scan, could only scan the head (which had to be surrounded by a bag of water to reduce the range of dynamic x-rays), and could take hours to process the information for the radiologist to read! (Beckmann, 2006). Current CT scans produce three-dimensional (3D) images, take only minutes to obtain, scan any body part or organ, and have

64- to 356-slice capability! CT scans are further enhanced with the use of different contrast media, which localizes to particular image cuts, highlighting images for the interpreting radiologist.

Fast Facts

The higher the "slice number" of a CT scanner, the thinner the horizontal picture is. For example, a 128-slice CT scanner will take twice the number of pictures as a 64-slice scanner, providing a greater number of images for the radiologist and making it possible to identify even smaller pathology before it grows larger.

CT scans have grown in popularity over the years, with approximately 85 million scans taken annually in the United States and 63 million in Japan (Brenner, 2012; IMV, 2012; Tsushima, Taketomi-Takahashi, Takei, Otake, & Endo, 2010); although, in the United Kingdom, the average number of annual CT scans is a mere 3.4 million. The continued growth in the United States is fueled by the ever-present demand to decrease ED overcrowding, the demand for a quick path to diagnosis, faster implementation of treatment, reduced time in radiology and EDs, and facilitation of hospital admission that is often prompted by a CT scan. The use of CT scans for virtual colonoscopies and oncology treatment planning also adds to the increased use of this technology.

When patients come in for their scan, remember this event from the patient's perspective. It is always a time of stress regardless if they are an outpatient (*often pending a difficult diagnosis and already worried about the impact such bad news would have on their family*), an inpatient (*scan results could mean complication of hospital course*), or an ED patient (*does their acute abdominal pain mean they'll need surgery?*). A patient rarely comes to the CT scanner without an element of extreme worry about what the scan may reveal and ultimately mean for their state of health. The nurse caring for this patient must focus on the "patient behind the image" and guide each patient through the experience. Providing for their privacy and utilizing therapeutic touch, eye contact, and listening to what is being said (or *not* being said) will make the experience ultimately less stressful for the patient, allow the technologist to obtain better images, and allow for a more accurate patient assessment for the nurse.

Fast Facts

Each CT table has a weight limit and a bore girth limit. To maintain patient dignity, weigh and measure the patient prior to placing the patient onto the CT table. When moving larger patients, mobilize additional staff to assist and employ professional sensitivity as large patients often worry about falling from skinny tables or not fitting into small places. Treat the patient with respect and educate them regarding your decision-making process.

SCREENING

Perform an accurate and thorough patient assessment prior to each CT scan, even if the patient was recently scanned. Individual organizational policy will dictate what should be reviewed during the patient history and how the scan procedure may be altered based on information obtained during the patient pre-scan assessment. Conditions that may be considered are as follows:

- **Allergies**
  - A history of prior anaphylactic reaction to an allergen may place the patient at a higher risk of reacting to CT contrast media.
  - Shellfish/seafood allergy does *not* predispose a patient to a contrast media allergy.
  - A prior allergic reaction to contrast media is a serious finding and needs careful attention before the patient receives contrast in the future (see the premedication section).
- **Anxiety**
  - Provide a calm environment for all patients, and educate them on each step of the scan process as it is imperative for patients to be motionless during the CT scan.
  - Be professional and convey competence to patients.
- **Asthma**
  - Consider listening to breath sounds and identifying when the patient last used their rescue inhaler.
  - There may be an increased risk of intravenous (IV) contrast reaction in patients with asthma.
- **Breastfeeding**
  - It is considered safe for breastfeeding mothers to receive contrast. Less than 1% of iodinated contrast media administered to a mother is excreted through her breast

milk. Less than 1% of the contrast media in breast milk is absorbed into the infant's gastrointestinal tract (ACR, 2013; ACR, version 10.3, 2018).

- For mothers who would like more information, they can contact the Poison Control Center at (800) 222-1222 for the latest information on contrast media and breastfeeding.

- **Cardiac status**
  - Take care when administering contrast media to patients with a cardiac history, including angina, hypertension (treated with medication), congestive heart failure, severe aortic stenosis, primary pulmonary hypertension, or cardiomyopathy.
  - Decreasing the volume or osmolality of contrast may increase patient safety.
  - .Refer to "physiological effects of contrast" for more information.

- **Devices**
  - Identify and, if possible, remove metal from the body as it will create "scatter" on the image: It will distort the images being interpreted by the radiologist.
  - Remove any types of metal in the area of the body to be scanned (i.e., body piercings, jewelry, hearing aids, etc.).
  - Insulin pumps, medication pumps, and other medical devices should be thoroughly investigated and discussed with the CT technologist and radiologist.

- **Dehydration**
  - Dehydration may increase the risk of nephrotoxicity in patients with impaired renal function, multiple myeloma, sickle cell disease, gout, homocystinuria, and so forth.
  - Blood urea nitrogen (BUN) > 20 mg/dL may indicate the need for hydration before/after receiving IV iodinated contrast media.

- **Hypertension**
  - Patients who receive medication to treat hypertension are at increased risk of contrast-induced nephrotoxicity.

- **Hyperthyroidism**
  - Graves' disease, Plummer disease (toxic multinodular goiter), and toxic adenoma may predispose a patient to thyrotoxicosis 4 to 6 weeks after receiving IV iodinated contrast.

- **Metformin**
  - Metformin is excreted unchanged from the kidneys and causes increased lactic acid production from the intestines. IV contrast is also excreted through the kidneys, and together there may be an increased workload on the kidneys.
  - Liver dysfunction, alcohol abuse, cardiac failure, infection, sepsis, or any muscle ischemia increase the risk of lactic acidosis occurring in these patients.

- Patients may be advised by their doctor to omit metformin from their regime for 48 hours post IV contrast administration.
- **Multiple myeloma**
  - May develop irreversible renal failure following administration of high-osmolality contrast media, especially if the patient is dehydrated.
- **Pheochromocytoma**
  - High-osmolality contrast media may increase the serum catecholamine levels and result in hypertensive crisis, while nonionic contrast media may have no influence on serum catecholamine levels (Bessell-Browne & O'Malley, 2007).
- **Pregnancy**
  - Iodinated contrast media crosses the placenta and enters the fetus.
  - The risk of IV contrast and exposure to CT radiation should be thoroughly explained to the pregnant mother by the physician, and informed consent signed prior to the procedure.
- **Renal insufficiency**
  - Increased serum creatinine level (>1.3 mg/dL) or decreased glomerular filtration rate (<59 mL/min) may indicate a risk for contrast-induced nephrotoxicity (CIN).
  - Lab work should be within 24 hours for the typical inpatient or ED patient. Some organizations use the 4- to 6-week time period for lab values with outpatients.
  - Emergent situations (stroke, trauma, etc.) may necessitate obtaining the CT scan without waiting for lab results, per organization policy.
  - Predisposing factors for CIN could include:
    - Age >60 years old
    - History of renal disease
      - Kidney transplant
      - Single kidney
      - Renal cancer
      - Renal surgery
      - Proteinuria
    - Diabetes mellitus
    - Taking a medication containing metformin (used to treat diabetes; may also be used by some physicians in the treatment of polycystic ovary syndrome)
    - Dehydration (BUN > 20 mg/dL)
    - Hypertension (receiving medication for treatment)
    - Multiple contrasted studies in less than a 24- to 48-hour period
- **Sickle cell disease**
  - There is some belief that IV contrast can promote sickle cell crisis.

PATIENT EDUCATION ON CT IMAGING

Begin educating the patient having a CT scan at the point of introduction and explanation of your role in their care. This might be their first experience having a CT scan or their first experience with a particular type of contrast. Help them feel welcome and safe in your department and explain what you are going to do *before* you do it. Take the time to answer their questions and involve patients in their care as much as possible.

- Teach your patients about:
  - Scan table and scanner
    - Movement of the table and scanner
    - Breath-holding instructions
    - Proper position for the patient to be in during the scan
    - That staff can see them, even though the patient is alone in the room
  - Injection
    - Purpose of IV contrast
    - Position of extremity (with peripheral IV placed)
    - Possible sensations which occur during injection
  - Post scan
    - Seek advice from their ordering physician regarding avoidance of metformin-containing medications for 48 hours post contrast injection
    - Importance of hydration post contrast (if received IV contrast)
    - Possibility of mild gastrointestinal (GI) symptoms (if received PO contrast)
    - Contact "911" for respiratory distress or medical emergency
    - Contact MD for mild allergic-type reactions up to 7 days post IV contrast
    - When scan will be interpreted by the radiologist and results to the ordering physician

SPECIAL CONSIDERATIONS

CT technology is useful in other areas of healthcare such as dentistry, virtual colonography, radiation therapy, PET scans, and areas outside of healthcare where industrial CT scanning may assist with fields such as museum artifact conservation, engineering applications, law enforcement, veterinary care, and industrial metrology.

- Dental CT scans provide 3D images that are used in special situations such as diagnosing pathology (or tumors) and surgical planning.
- Virtual CT colonoscopy has less risk, costs less, and is less invasive than a conventional colonoscopy, although it does expose the patient to radiation, and if pathology is identified, the patient will need to undergo a conventional colonoscopy for treatment.
- PET scans are nuclear medicine scans and CT scans that are superimposed on each other, which provide the radiologist with images that identify molecular activity within the body as well as interpretable images.
- CT scanning assists veterinarians in diagnosis.
- Industrial metrology utilizes CT technology in ensuring high quality output.

References

American College of Radiology. (2013). *Manual on contrast media, version 9*. Retrieved from http://www.acr.org/Quality-Safety/Resources/Contrast-Manual

American College of Radiology. (2018). *Manual on contrast media, version v10.3*. https://www.acr.org/Clinical-Resources/Contrast-Manual

Beckmann, E. (2006). CT scanning in the early days. *British Journal of Radiology, 79*, 5–8. doi:10.1259/bjr/29444122

Bessell-Browne, R., & O'Malley, M. E. (2007). CT of pheochromocytoma and paraganglioma: Risk of adverse events with I.V. administration of nonionic contrast material. *American Journal of Roentgenology, 188*(4), 970–974. doi:10.2214/AJR.06.0827

Brenner, D. J. (2012). Minimizing medically unwarranted computed tomography scans. *Annals of the International Commission on Radiological Protection, 41*(3–4), 161–169. doi:10.1016/j.icrp.2012.06.004

International Marketing Ventures. (2012). *2012 CT market outlook report*. Des Plaines, IL: International Marketing Ventures.

Tsushima, Y., Taketomi-Takahashi, A., Takei, H., Otake, H., & Endo, K. (2010). Radiation exposure from CT examinations in Japan. *BMC Medical Imaging, 10*, 24. Retrieved from http://www.biomedcentral.com/1471-2342/10/24

11

Iodinated Contrast Media Basics

Ana Davis

Contrast media enhances CT images read by the radiologist and results in a more accurate identification of internal structures and pathology. Contrast may be administered orally, intravenously, and/or rectally. Careful screening of patients should occur prior to the administration of any type of contrast.

In this chapter, you will discover:

1. Screening of patient prior to receiving contrast
2. Different types of contrast media
3. Physiologic effects of intravenous (IV) iodinated contrast

CONTRAST

Common types of contrast for CT scan:

- **Oral**
Most institutions require that the patient fasts for at least 3 hours prior to the scan. Oral contrast is indicated to help diagnose problems in esophagus, stomach, and bowels.
    - Barium sulfate
        - Contraindicated if bowel obstruction or perforation is suspected, or if patient may go to surgery after the CT scan.

- Iodinated water-soluble contrast
  - Water-soluble contrast media can be made with low-osmolality contrast media (LOCM) or high-osmolality contrast media (HOCM).
  - Diluted with water for CT scans.
- Water
  - Plain water may be used as an oral contrast for certain exams.

- **Rectal**
  - Iodinated water-soluble contrast mixed with water, given via enema just prior to scanning.

- **Intravenous iodinated contrast media**
  - Injected through a patent IV line, it opacifies the vessels in its flow path, allowing the visualization of internal structures until significant hemodilution occurs. The contrast media subsequently flows toward the extravascular compartments, where it is absorbed by normal and abnormal tissues in the body and the brain. Finally, it is excreted unchanged through the kidneys by glomerular filtration.
  - Three primary forms of contrast exist:
    - HOCM; the oldest agent with limited use
    - LOCM; water-soluble and most commonly used
    - Nonionic or iso-osmolar contrast media (IOCM); is water-soluble
  - IV CT contrast should be warmed to body temperature prior to administration to decrease the viscosity and promote safer injection.
  - Always verify IV patency (peripheral or central lines) by following manufacturer and organizational policy (venous backflow, easily flushed with palpable thrill, painless insertion site, visual image of central venous catheter tip, etc.).

Fast Facts

To prevent an air embolism, perform a double safety check when connecting the tubing from the power injector to the patient's IV: Survey the entire length of the tubing with your eyes, observing for air just prior to connecting the injector tubing to the patient's intravenous line, and look for a drop of contrast protruding from the tip of the tubing.

PHYSIOLOGICAL EFFECTS OF IODINATED CONTRAST INJECTION

- **Gastrointestinal tract effects following IV contrast injection**
  - Nausea, vomiting, diarrhea, cramping
  - Some patients may "taste" a metallic flavor

- **Pulmonary effects following IV contrast injection**
  - Bronchoconstriction may occur due to histamine release as contrast is identified as a foreign body in the bloodstream.

- **Renal effects following IV contrast injection**
  - Healthy kidneys will excrete contrast in 2 to 4 hours; impaired kidneys (reduced glomerular filtration rate [GFR], elevated creatinine, elevated blood urea nitrogen [BUN]) may take several days to excrete contrast.
  - It can take up to a week for a serum creatinine to return to normal after a patient receives IV contrast.
  - Patients with diabetes and preexisting renal insufficiency are at greatest risk of nephrotoxicity.
  - Increased risk of contrast-induced nephrotoxicity (CIN) in patients who have received contrast within the previous 24 to 48 hours.

Fast Facts

Anuric end-stage chronic kidney disease patients can receive IV iodinated contrast. Their kidneys are no longer functioning, and it will be cleared with dialysis. Emergent dialysis is not necessary, but some recommend dialysis within 24 hours of contrast injection. Take care with oliguric patients; there is a belief they may be converted to anuric patients after receiving IV iodinated contrast media.

- **Thyroid effects following IV contrast injection**
  - Iodine in contrast agents can stimulate an acute overproduction of thyroid hormone (thyrotoxicosis) in patients with hyperthyroidism, but this is a rare complication.
- **Vascular effects following IV contrast injection**
  - Fluid shifts from the tissues to the veins because contrast has higher osmolality than blood (contrast is heavier than blood, fluid from cells goes back into the veins to thin the blood).

- Red blood cells shrink because the water is removed from the cell (crenation) to help balance blood plasma–contrast solution.
  - This crenation of the red blood cell (RBC) causes their shape to change and thus an inability to float through the capillaries with ease and ultimately decreases oxygenation to the tissues, causing pain—this can be harmful to patients with sickle cell anemia.
  - Thrombosis or ischemia may occur, especially in the brain or myocardium.
- Peripheral vasodilation that may make the patient feel "warmth" or "hot flash."
- Localized vasodilation at injection site may feel like a "burn" that calms down after a few seconds.
- Transient hypotension.
- Care should be taken with compromised patients, including those with aortic stenosis, severe coronary artery disease, and so forth.

Fast Facts

Power injectors force contrast through the body at precision speed to be expertly timed with the radiation scanning of the CT. Remember the equivalent injection rates of the power injector: (power injector rate) 1 mL/second is equivalent to 3,600 mL/hour (IV pump rate)

2 mL/second is equivalent to 7,200 mL/hour

3 mL/second is equivalent to 10,800 mL/hour

4 mL/second is equivalent to 14,400 mL/hour

5 mL/second is equivalent to 18,000 mL/hour

PATIENT SCREENING

Risk Factors
- Renal disease
- Diabetes mellitus
- Hypertension
- Age >60
- History of allergy or multiple allergies
- Asthma/bronchospasm

- Anxiety
- Systemic lupus erythematosus
- Dehydration
- Anemia

Venous Access

- Poor venous competency increases the risk of extravasation; antecubital or large forearm vein is recommended for injections.

Current Medications That Can Increase Risk of Adverse Reactions

- Beta-blockers
- Ca channel blockers
- Metformin hydrochloride
- Interleukin-2 (IL-2) immunotherapy
- Nephrotoxic drugs

Laboratory Values

- Normal values: eGFR >59 mL/min/1.73 m^2, BUN 6 to 20 mg/dL

PREINJECTION VERIFICATION ("TIME OUT")

Prior to each injection of contrast, each organization must have a policy that directs all present staff to *stop* and verify key information about the patient to be scanned. At a minimum, the following should be included in this "time out":

- Two patient identifiers
- Review of the provider's order for scan
- Verify the correct body region to be scanned
- Reconciled allergies and other risks
- Correct contrast; dose and rate of injection

It is crucial for the nurse or technologist who performs the injection to be present for the "time out" before approving the start of the contrast injection.

PATIENT EDUCATION ON IV CONTRAST INJECTION

Patient education should begin at the moment you are introducing yourself and explaining your role in their care. For some patients, this may be their first CT scan or perhaps their first experience with a particular type of contrast. Help them feel welcome and safe in your department, and explain what you are going to do *before* you do it. Take the time to answer questions and involve patients in their care as much as possible.

- Teach your patients about:
  - Injection
    - Purpose of IV contrast
    - Position of extremity (with peripheral IV placed)
    - Possible sensations that may occur during injection
      - "Hot flash" anywhere from their throat, stomach, genital region
      - May feel as though they are urinating on themselves
  - Scan table and scanner
    - Movement of the table and scanner
    - Breath-holding instructions when applicable
    - Proper position during the scan, and to avoid moving after scout scans done
    - That staff can see and hear them, even though they are alone in the room
  - Post scan
    - Seeking advice from their ordering physician regarding avoidance of metformin-containing medications for 48 hours post contrast injection
    - Importance of hydration post contrast (if received IV contrast)
    - Possibility of mild gastrointestinal [GI] symptoms (if received PO contrast) or headache (if received IV contrast)
    - Contacting "911" for respiratory distress or medical emergency
    - Contacting MD for mild allergic-type reactions that can occur up to 7 days post IV contrast
    - Finding out when results will be interpreted by radiologist and available to ordering provider

Additional Resource

American College of Radiology. (2020). *Manual on contrast media*. Retrieved from https://www.acr.org/Clinical-Resources/Contrast-Manual

12

Iodinated Contrast Adverse Events

Ana Davis

Allergic or adverse reactions can occur at any time and to any type of contrast. A known history of an adverse reaction needs to be fully investigated, and a careful plan of care must be created for the patient prior to the administration of contrast. If a patient experiences a reaction to contrast, the imaging team must be able to react quickly to provide appropriate care to the patient.

In this chapter, you will discover:

1. Identifying types of reactions
2. Emergency treatment of reactions
3. Treatment of extravasation
4. Pretreatment for prior contrast reactions

IODINATED CONTRAST ADVERSE EVENTS

CT contrast risks have diminished over the years due to changes in its formulation and improved knowledge regarding its use. Adverse events range from intravenous (IV) extravasations to allergic reactions. For safe patient care in the CT scan setting, follow the steps discussed in this chapter.

Allergic IV CT contrast reactions may occur immediately or be delayed by up to 7 days. Typically, the more severe the reaction, the quicker the symptoms begin; if the patient begins to exhibit symptoms before the scan is complete, mobilize a response team immediately, as the patient is likely to progress to anaphylaxis quickly. Patients may experience a wide variety of contrast events requiring observation, treatment, and education.

People with asthma have 1.2 to 2.5 times the risk of such reactions than the general population. In addition, when the reactions occur, they are more likely to be severe. Patients with allergies, including hay fever, are 1.5 to 3 times more likely to have an adverse reaction to iodinated contrast media (ICM) than other people.

- *Mild reactions* appear self-limited without evidence of progression.
  - Allergic signs or symptoms include:
    - Urticaria/pruritus
    - Cutaneous edema
    - Itchy or scratchy throat
    - Nasal congestion
    - Sneezing, conjunctivitis, rhinorrhea
  - Physiologic signs or symptoms include:
    - Nausea or vomiting (commonly seen)
    - Transient flushing, warmth, chills
    - Headache, dizziness, anxiety, altered taste
    - Mild hypertension
    - Vasovagal reaction that resolves without treatment
- *Moderate reactions* are more pronounced and may progress to a more severe reaction if treatment is delayed.
  - Allergic signs or symptoms include:
    - Diffuse urticaria or pruritus
    - Diffuse erythema with stable vital signs
    - Facial edema without dyspnea
    - Throat tightness or hoarseness without dyspnea
    - Wheezing or bronchospasm with mild or no hypoxia
  - Physiologic reactions:
    - Protracted nausea or vomiting
    - Hypertensive urgency
    - Isolated chest pain
    - Vasovagal reaction that responds to required treatment
- *Severe reactions* are often life-threatening and may result in permanent injury or death if not managed immediately and appropriately.
  - Patient condition may quickly progress to cardiopulmonary arrest
  - Pulmonary edema, although rare, can occur in patients with impaired cardiac function

- Allergic life-threatening reactions:
  - Diffuse edema with or without facial edema causing dyspnea
  - Diffuse erythema with hypotension
  - Laryngeal edema with stridor and/or hypoxia
  - Wheezing or bronchospasm with significant hypoxia
  - Anaphylactic shock with hypotension and tachycardia
- Physiologic life-threatening reactions:
  - Vasovagal reaction resistant to treatment
  - Arrhythmia
  - Seizure
  - Hypertensive crisis

- **Reaction Management**
  - If you suspect a patient is having a reaction, stop the injection immediately, and do *not* remove the IV; it may be needed later for treatment.
  - Call for additional personnel to assist and perform a rapid patient assessment with vital signs.
  - Interventions will depend upon your patient's signs and symptoms, but could include the following:
    - Monitor vital signs (heart rate, respiratory rate, blood pressure, oximetry, capnography, electrocardiogram, etc.)
    - IV fluids (hypotension, anaphylaxis, hypoglycemia)
    - Administer oxygen (bronchospasm, laryngeal edema, hypo/hypertension, pulmonary edema, seizures)
    - Access patient's medical history, medication list, allergies, weight
    - Position for rescue
      - Elevate the head of the bed (dyspnea, pulmonary edema)
      - Trendelenburg (hypotension)
      - Position patient on their side (seizures)
  - Medications for treatment may include:
    - Diphenhydramine (hives)
    - Epinephrine (progressive hives, diffuse erythema, bronchospasm, laryngeal edema)
    - Beta agonist inhaler (bronchospasm)
    - Atropine (hypotension, bradycardia)
    - Labetalol (hypertension)
    - Nitroglycerin (hypertension)
    - Furosemide (hypertension, pulmonary edema)
    - Morphine (pulmonary edema)

- ❏ Lorazepam (seizures)
- ❏ Dextrose 50% (hypoglycemia)
- ❏ Glucagon (hypoglycemia)
⇒ Refer to current advanced cardiac life support (ACLS) guidelines, rescue protocols, and your organizational policies

- **Allergy Premedication (Iodinated Contrast Media)**

For patients with prior adverse reactions to IV iodinated contrast, premedication will be ordered prior to them receiving IV iodinated contrast for scans. While there are different prescriber preferences with the premedication regime, realize the importance of antihistamines. The maximum prophylactic benefit of corticosteroids occurs minimally 6 to 13 hours after the first dose is administered. After identifying an "at-risk" patient from a history of prior contrast reaction, the current recommendation from the 2020 American College of Radiology (ACR) Contrast Manual for premedication regimen is:

Elective Studies
Option #1
1. Prednisone: 50 mg by mouth at 13 hours, 7 hours, and 1 hour before contrast injection

and

2. Diphenhydramine: 50 mg by mouth, IV, or intramuscular (IM) 1 hour prior to contrast injection

Option #2
1. Methylprednisolone: 32 mg by mouth at 12 hours and 2 hours prior to contrast injection

and

2. Diphenhydramine: 50 mg by mouth, IV, or IM 1 hour prior to contrast injection

Fast Facts

- IV corticosteroids are not effective when administered less than 4 hours prior to contrast injection.
- Careful blood glucose monitoring should occur in diabetic patients who receive corticosteroids.

Emergent Studies

Option #1

1. Methylprednisolone sodium succinate: 40 mg IV or hydrocortisone sodium succinate 200 mg IV immediately and every 4 hours until contrast injection administered

and

2. Diphenhydramine: 50 mg IV one hour prior to contrast injection (regimen usually 4 to 5 hours in duration)

Option #2

1. Dexamethasone sodium sulfate 7.5 mg IV every 4 hours until contrast injection administered
2. Diphenhydramine: 50 mg IV one hour prior to contrast injection (regimen usually 4 to 5 hours in duration)

Option #3

1. Omit steroids
2. Diphenhydramine: 50 mg IV one hour prior to contrast injection

Pediatric Patients

1. Prednisone: 0.5 to 0.7 mg/kg by mouth (up to 50 mg) given 13, 7, and 1 hour prior to contrast injection
2. Diphenhydramine: 1.25 mg/kg by mouth (up to 50 mg) 1 hour prior to contrast injection

EXTRAVASATION OF IODINATED CONTRAST MEDIA (CT)

Every patient who receives IV contrast is at risk of extravasation; therefore, it is imperative to work diligently to prevent it.

- **Prevention of extravasations include:**
  - Optimal IV placement for patient condition (most appropriate gauge, site) and injection rate for the study to be conducted.
  - Verifying IV patency prior to injection (follow manufacturer and organizational guidelines, which normally include venous backflow and forceful saline flush).
  - Educating patient about expectations (straight and motionless arms, hot flash feeling, etc.).
  - Maintaining hyperfocus on the patient during actual injection.
    - Remain in the scan room with the patient, if possible; maintain manual contact at the IV insertion site monitoring the thrill; be prepared to immediately stop the injection if extravasation occurs.

Fast Facts

If you must monitor an IV power injection from the CT control room, keep your eyes on the patient at all times until the injection is complete. In most cases, as an extravasation begins, the patient will flinch, curl their fingers or toes, and you will hear them scream in pain, giving you advance notice and allowing you to stop the injection and minimize the severity of the extravasation.

- *Patients who are at increased risk for extravasations* include those who
  - Cannot communicate adequately;
    - Are at extremes of age (elderly/infants or children); and
    - Are with altered consciousness.
  - Are severely ill, injured, debilitated, or uncooperative for any reason
  - Have abnormal circulation to the extremity, including:
    - Peripheral/diabetic vascular disease
    - Stroke
    - Raynaud's disease
    - Venous thrombosis or insufficiency
    - Compromised venous/lymphatic drainage in the extremity used for IV injection
    - Radiation therapy
    - Extensive surgery in the limb in which the injection will be done (lymph node dissection, vein graft harvesting, etc.)
  - Emaciation/cachexia
  - Marked peripheral edema
  - Have IV sites located in the:
    - Hand
    - Wrist
    - Foot
    - Ankle
  - Have IV sites that were:
    - Placed longer than 24 hours
    - Difficult to cannulate
    - Placed by an ambulance crew or during a code situation
    - Already used for multiple power injections
    - Placed in the upper arm with ample loose tissue
- *Treatment of extravasation* (no clear best practice)
  - Immediately stop the infusion of the contrast media at the first sign of extravasation.

- Notify the physician/radiologist.
- Elevate the affected extremity above the level of the heart to decrease capillary hydrostatic pressure.
- To relieve the pain apply:
  - *Dry*, warm compresses that may promote vasodilation and improve absorption and blood flow; or
  - *Dry*, cold compresses that may relieve pain at the injection site.
- May attempt injection of corticosteroids after consultation with provider
- Document the following information in the patient's medical record:
  - The location of infiltration (if possible, measure the size and extent and/or girth of the area affected); and
  - The type and amount of contrast medium.
  - The treatment rendered
- Assess the extremity involved for any of the following:
  - Redness
  - Blisters
  - Ulceration
  - Firmness
  - Changes in temperature, movement, or sensation (ACR, 2020)
- Patients must be given clear instructions for follow-up, which include seeking medical help for the development of ulcers, worsening pain or swelling, or change in sensation or circulation.
- Verbal nurse-to-nurse report (handoff) should occur and be documented in the medical record for inpatients and ED patients after contrast extravasation.
- Good nursing practice includes a follow-up call 24 hours post extravasation to assess patient condition and document in patient's record.

Reference

American College of Radiology. (2020). *Manual on contrast media*. Retrieved from https://www.acr.org/Clinical-Resources/Contrast-Manual

13

MRI Basics and Magnet Safety

Velecia Marston

MRI uses magnetic and electromagnetic fields, which create a resonance effect of hydrogen atoms. The electromagnetic emission created by these atoms is registered and processed by the computer to produce images of body structures.

In this chapter, you will discover:

1. Screening for magnet safety
2. Use of MRI scan technology
3. Essential patient education

MAGNETIC RESONANCE IMAGING

In 1974, the first patent was obtained for an MRI scanner, and it was not until 1977 that the first patient was scanned. It took nearly 5 hours to produce just one image (that first MRI scanner is now housed in the Smithsonian Institution!). Fast forward to 2018, where there were 24.7 MRI scans per 1,000 people in Chili, 118.9 MRI scans per 1,000 people in the United States, and 143.4 scans per 1,000 people in Germany (OECD, 2019).

MRI provides an unparalleled view inside of the human body by using strong magnetic fields and radio waves. Both work together to produce cross-sectional images of organs and internal structures of the body. The MRI detects the signal, which varies depending on the water content and local magnetic properties of the particular body part being imaged, and thus, different tissues or substances can be distinguished from one another in the resulting scan. An electrical current is passed through wires in a coil, creating a temporary magnetic field around the patient's body. The radio waves are sent and received from within the machine, and these signals are used to produce the digital image of the body part being scanned.

Fast Facts

Common units of measure for magnets are tesla and gauss (1 tesla = 10,000 gauss). Most MRI magnets used today are 0.5 to 3 tesla (5,000–30,000 gauss). Some research is being done with 10.5 tesla. Compare that to the earth's natural magnetic pull that is measured at a mere 0.5 gauss!

MRI is valuable for imaging and diagnosing:

- Multiple sclerosis
- Tumors of the pituitary gland, brain, bone
- Infections of the brain, spine, joints
- Ligaments injuries
- Joint injuries (shoulder, knee, back)
- Tendonitis
- Early stages of strokes
- Cysts

MAGNET SAFETY AND SCREENING

Considering the intense magnetic pull of the MRI, the MRI personnel must be diligent to protect the safety of whoever may come near it. Both paid personnel and visitors must be screened for magnet safety, questioning metal inside of the body or outside of the body. The list is extensive and cannot be fully covered in this text; however, a brief overview will be discussed. A person's simple attestation, "They are safe to go near the magnet," is insufficient: Each person must be fully screened for magnet safety prior to admittance to the MR environment (Kanal, 2013).

Fast Facts

For the latest information on MRI safety and practice guidance, visit www.mrisafety.com.

- **Personnel Magnet Safety and Screening**
  - Each organization must have an MR medical director as well as an MR safety director who maintains the updated safety structure for the department. Initial orientation and annual competency for those directly involved with MR patient care must include appropriate documentation of education and attendance at a 1-hour live lecture or recorded presentation (Kanal, 2013).
  - Staff who provide care for patients near the magnet must be screened annually for magnet safety, and documentation must be maintained. They should be screened for the same safety risks as the patients, and such documentation should be kept on file.
  - Prior to entering the MR scanner, staff must remove all metal from their body including:
    - Wallets (containing bank/ID cards with metallic strips)
    - Pagers, cell phones, watches, pens, keys, nail clippers, jewelry, hair decorations
    - Pocket knife, law enforcement weapons, tools
    - Any metal object will become a dangerous item near the magnet!

- **Patient Magnet Safety and Screening**
  - Patients should be screened for magnet safety by two qualified MR personnel prior to routine scans, and by one qualified MR personnel prior to an emergency scan.
  - Unconscious patients who have no history available should minimally have orbital x-rays obtained to screen for metal fragments prior to MRI.
  - Ask patients the same question in different ways to uncover terminology differences that could be a safety hazard for the patient (i.e., pacemaker vs. implanted device).
  - Identify if patients have any of the following:
    - Metal objects in the eye (shavings, slivers, etc.)

- Any type of electronic, mechanical, or magnetic implant
- Aneurysm clips
- Cardiac pacemaker or defibrillator
- Stimulator (bio-stimulator, neuro-stimulator, spinal cord, bone growth, etc.)
- Internal wires or electrodes
- Cochlear or other otologic implant
- Drug-infusion pump (insulin, chemo, pain medicine, etc.)
- Any prosthesis of any kind
- Implanted valves, joints, rods, pins, devices, coils, filters, stents, clips, staples, shunts, springs, wires, mesh, seeds, plates, dental work, etc.
- Metal object (BB, shrapnel, bullet, etc.)
- Vascular access (port, peripherally inserted central catheter [PICC], etc.)
- Tissue expander (i.e., breast)
- Removable or permanent dental piece, denture, or partial plate
- Electronic monitoring device
- Body piercings or implants
- Wig or hair implants
- Tattoos or permanent makeup (newly placed)
- Intrauterine device (IUD), diaphragm, or vaginal pessary
- Hearing aid
- Any piece of anything that they were not born with!

- Additionally, the MR staff will need to carefully assess patients who have:
  - Endotracheal or tracheotomy tubes
  - Central lines, Swan-Ganz catheter, arterial line transducers, etc.
  - Foley catheter with a temperature sensor and/or a metal clamp
  - Esophageal or rectal probes
  - Guidewires

- Prior to entering the MR scanner, patients will be asked to:
  - Use the restroom, if necessary.
  - Wear earplugs or headphones.
  - Remove jewelry, hair decorations, removable denture plates, hearing aids, eyeglasses, watch, pager, wallets, purses, cell phones, select body piercings, and clothing with metal.

PATIENT HISTORY AND SCREENING

In addition to screening patients for magnet safety, staff must screen patients for medical history, renal issues, and their ability to comply with the MRI procedure. Prior to positioning the patient on the MRI scan table, determine the following:

- Previous MRI scan or other imaging performed
- Concern for claustrophobia (sedation, someone to drive patient home, etc.)
- History of eye injury (when, type, treatment, etc.)
- Current medication list
- Medication allergies (source, reaction, treatment, premedication, etc.)
- Contrast allergies (type of contrast, reaction, etc.)
- History of asthma, respiratory disease, hypertension, cancer, seizures, diabetes, liver disease, renal disease of any type, anemia, sickle cell anemia, etc. (determined specifics of each illness)
- Pregnancy screening (last normal menstrual period [LNMP], pregnancy test results, fertility treatments, etc.)
- Breastfeeding

PATIENT EDUCATION ON MRI

- Teach your patients about:
  - Scan table and scanner
    - Earplugs/headphones to protect their hearing from the sound of the MRI scanner in motion
    - Movement of the table and scanner
    - Breath-holding instructions
    - Proper position for the patient to be in during the scan
    - That staff can see them, even though patient is alone in the room
    - The patient role in image acquisition (holding still, following instructions, etc.)
  - Injection
    - Purpose of intravenous (IV) contrast
    - Possible sensation that occurs during injection
  - Post scan
    - When results will be interpreted by radiologist

Fast Facts

Help your patient to feel welcomed and safe in your department. Explain what you are going to do *before* you do it. Take the time to answer their questions and involve patients in their care as much as possible. The more relaxed the patient is, the more cooperative they can be and the better the imaging will be!

References

Kanal, E., Barkovich, J., Bell, C., Borgstede, J., Bradley, W., Froelich, J., & Hernandez, D. (2013). ACR guidance document on MR safe practice. *Journal of Magnetic Resonance Imaging, 37*(3), 501–530. doi:10.1002/jmri.24011

OECD. (2019). *Magnetic resonance imaging (MRI) exams (indicator).* doi:10.1787/1d89353f-en

14

MRI Contrast Media Basics

Ana Davis

MRI contrast agents work by altering the local magnetic field of the tissue being imaged. The different types of contrast agents may be administered by oral and/or intravenous (IV) routes.

In this chapter, you will discover:

1. The screening items needed prior to patient receiving contrast
2. The different types of MRI contrast media
3. Emergency treatment of contrast reaction

CONTRAST

MRI contrast agents alter the local magnetic field of the tissue being imaged. The different types may include:

- Oral
  - Ultra low-dose/dilute barium sulfate (i.e., VoLumen)
  - Fruit juice (pineapple, blueberry)
  - Water
  - Methylcellulose
  - Polyethylene glycol (ACR, 2020)
- IV
  - Gadolinium is a paramagnetic metal ion that moves differently within a magnetic field. Gadolinium-based contrast agents

(GBCAs) are extremely well-tolerated and the occurrence of adverse reactions is lower than those that occur with iodinated contrast media.

- GBCAs are administered at room temperature per manufacturer guidelines, and should *not* be warmed prior to IV injection.
- When injecting GBCAs for IV contrast, observe the same safety steps as with CT IV contrast injections (see Chapter 11, Iodinated Contrast Media Basics).

PATIENT HISTORY AND SCREENING

Obtain patient's information regarding the following:

- Allergies (source, reaction, treatment, premedication, etc.)
- Current medications
- Metabolic acidosis
- Immunosuppression
- Liver disease
- Age > 60 years old
- Acute or chronic renal disease (dialysis, renal surgery, single kidney, cancer)
- Multiple myeloma
- Systemic lupus erythematosus
- Pregnancy screening (last normal menstrual period [LMP], pregnancy test results, fertility treatments, etc.)
- Estimated glomerular filtration rate (eGFR) <60 mL/min: Lab work should be within 48 hours to 6 weeks depending on comorbidities (ACR, 2020)

PREINJECTION VERIFICATION ("TIME OUT")

Prior to each injection of contrast, each organization must have a policy that directs all present staff to *stop* and verify key information about the patient to be scanned. At a minimum, the following should be included in this "time out":

- Two patient identifiers
- Review of the provider's order for scan
- Verification of the correct body region to be scanned
- Reconciled allergies and other risks
- Correct contrast, dose, and rate of injection

It is crucial for the nurse or technologist who performs the injection to be present for the "time out" before approving the start of the contrast injection.

IV PATENCY

- Optimal IV placement for patient condition (most appropriate gauge, site) and injection rate for the study to be conducted.
- Follow manufacturer and organizational guidelines to verify IV patency, which normally include venous backflow and forceful saline flush.

Fast Facts

To prevent an air embolism, perform a double safety check when connecting the tubing from the power injector to the patient's IV: Survey the entire length of the tubing with your eyes, observing for air just prior to connecting the injector tubing to the patient's intravenous line and look for a drop of contrast protruding from the tip of the tubing.

EXTRAVASATION

Many MRI scans utilizing IV gadolinium are hand injected, and therefore, the risk of extravasation is small, as the close monitoring of the injection should prevent most tissue damage from an infiltrate of gadolinium.

ADVERSE EVENTS

Acute adverse reactions to GBCAs are similar to those of iodinated contrast (see Chapter 12, Iodinated Contrast Adverse Events)

- Most reactions to the contrast administration are mild and physiological
  - Nausea/vomiting
  - Headache/dizziness/altered taste
  - Coldness, warmth, pain, or paresthesia at the injection site

- Allergic reactions include:
  - Rash
  - Hives
  - Urticaria/pruritus
  - Bronchospasm
  - Anaphylactoid
- Nephrogenic Systemic Fibrosis
  - Poorly functioning kidneys are not able to excrete gadolinium from the body
  - As a result, excessive fibrous tissue begins to grow on the eyes, skin, joints, and internal organs
  - For more information: www.fda.gov/Drugs/DrugSafety/ ucm223966.htm; https://www.fda.gov/drugs/drug-safety-and -availability/fda-drug-safety-communication-new-warnings -using-gadolinium-based-contrast-agents-patients-kidney

Fast Facts

MRI GBCA adverse reactions and treatment are similar to those of iodinated media. If a patient decompensates while in the MRI scanner, immediately *begin medical interventions while the patient is actively being moved out of the magnet area.* A preestablished, magnetically safe resuscitative area must be designated within the radiology department. Mock codes should be practiced and include preservation of magnet safety.

Reaction Management

- If you suspect a patient is having a reaction, do *not* remove the IV (you may need it later!)
- Call for additional personnel to assist and perform a rapid patient assessment with vital signs
- Interventions will depend upon your patient's signs and symptoms, but could include the following:
  - Monitor vital signs (heart rate, respiratory rate, blood pressure, oximetry, capnography, electrocardiogram, etc.)
  - IV fluids (hypotension, anaphylaxis, hypoglycemia)
  - Administer oxygen (bronchospasm, laryngeal edema, hypo/ hypertension, pulmonary edema, seizures)
  - Access patient's medical history, medication list, allergies, weight
  - Position for rescue
    - Elevate the head of the bed (dyspnea, pulmonary edema)

- ❏ Trendelenburg (hypotension)
- ❏ Position patient on their side (seizures)
- ■ Medications for treatment may include:
  - ❏ Diphenhydramine (hives)
  - ❏ Epinephrine (progressive hives, diffuse erythema, bronchospasm, laryngeal edema)
  - ❏ Beta agonist inhaler (bronchospasm)
  - ❏ Atropine (hypotension, bradycardia)
  - ❏ Labetalol (hypertension)
  - ❏ Nitroglycerin (hypertension)
  - ❏ Furosemide (hypertension, pulmonary edema)
  - ❏ Morphine (pulmonary edema)
  - ❏ Lorazepam (seizures)
  - ❏ Dextrose 50% (hypoglycemia)
  - ❏ Glucagon (hypoglycemia)
- ⇒ Refer to the current advanced cardiac life support (ACLS) guidelines, rescue protocols, and your organizational policies.

Allergy Premedication

For patients with prior adverse reactions to GBCAs, premedication will be ordered prior to them receiving GBCAs for scans. While there are different prescriber preferences with the premedication regime, it is important to realize the importance of antihistamines and that the maximum prophylactic benefit of corticosteroids occurs minimally 6 to 13 hours after the first dose is administered. After identifying an "at risk" patient from a history of prior contrast reaction, the current recommendation from the 2018 ACR Contrast Manual for premedication regimen is:

Elective Studies

Option #1

1. Prednisone: 50 mg by mouth at 13 hours, 7 hours, and 1 hour before contrast injection
   and
2. Diphenhydramine: 50 mg by mouth, IV, or intramuscular (IM) 1 hour prior to contrast injection

Option #2

1. Methylprednisolone: 32 mg by mouth at 12 hours and 2 hours prior to contrast injection
   and
2. Diphenhydramine: 50 mg by mouth, IV, or IM 1 hour prior to contrast injection

Emergent Studies

Option #1

1. Methylprednisolone sodium succinate: 40 mg IV or hydrocortisone sodium succinate 200 mg IV immediately and every 4 hours until contrast injection administered
   and
2. Diphenhydramine: 50 mg IV 1 hour prior to contrast injection (regimen usually 4–5 hours in duration)

Option #2

1. Dexamethasone sodium sulfate: 7.5 mg IV every 4 hours until contrast injection administered
2. Diphenhydramine: 50 mg IV 1 hour prior to contrast injection (regimen usually 4–5 hours in duration)

Option #3

1. Omit steroids
2. Diphenhydramine: 50 mg IV 1 hour prior to contrast injection

Pediatric Patients

1. Prednisone: 0.5 to 0.7 mg/kg by mouth (up to 50 mg) given at 13 hours, 7 hours, and 1 hour prior to contrast injection
2. Diphenhydramine: 1.25 mg/kg by mouth (up to 50 mg) 1 hour prior to contrast injection
   - Medications for treatment may include:
     - Diphenhydramine (hives)
     - Epinephrine (progressive hives, diffuse erythema, bronchospasm, laryngeal edema)
     - Beta agonist inhaler (bronchospasm)
     - Atropine (hypotension, bradycardia)
     - Labetalol (hypertension)
     - Nitroglycerin (hypertension)
     - Furosemide (hypertension, pulmonary edema)
     - Morphine (pulmonary edema)
     - Lorazepam (seizures)
     - Dextrose 50% (hypoglycemia)
     - Glucagon (hypoglycemia)
   - ⇒ Refer to current ACLS guidelines, rescue protocols, and your organizational policies.

PATIENT EDUCATION

- Teach your patients about:
  - Scan table and scanner
    - Earplugs and/or headphones to protect their hearing from the sound of the MRI scanner in motion
    - Movement of the table and scanner
    - Breath-holding instructions
    - Proper position for the patient to be in during the scan
    - That staff can see them, even though patient is alone in the room
    - Patient role in image acquisition (holding still, following instructions, etc.)
  - Injection
    - Purpose of IV contrast
    - Possible sensation that occurs during injection
  - Post scan
    - When results will be interpreted by radiologist

Reference

American College of Radiology. (2020). *Manual on contrast media*. Retrieved from https://www.acr.org/Clinical-Resources/Contrast-Manual

IV

Interventional Radiology

15

Neurointerventional Radiology Overview

Susan Deveikis and John P. Deveikis

The nervous system is vitally important for normal function of the individual. Neurointerventional procedures are minimally invasive treatments that can be used to treat neurovascular conditions. These procedures can complement or sometimes replace more traditional medical and surgical treatments. This chapter outlines concepts common to making neurointerventional procedures safer and more effective. Subsequent chapters will concentrate on neurointerventional treatments for cerebral ischemia and neurointerventional embolization procedures.

In this chapter, you will discover the importance of:

1. Good communication among all team members
2. Anticipating patient needs before, during, and after the procedure
3. Infection control during invasive procedures

COMMUNICATION

Communication is the key to providing high-quality and safe patient care. Every team member should be aware of the anticipated procedure and their role, and every team member should feel free to speak up if they see something is amiss. The operator (attending physician) should be the most informed person in the room, not the least informed, as they direct all the other team members. For example, the anesthesia team should be aware of their role during intracranial embolization. They should be prepared to make the patient immobile through paralytics and deep sedation and test the anesthetized patient periodically with a nerve stimulator to ensure adequate paralysis.

Prior to the procedure, a plan should be in place as to the anticipated disposition of the patient. For example, is the patient going to be an outpatient and do they have a designated driver? If the patient is to be admitted, will they need an ICU bed, monitored bed, or just floor status? Having this information allows for the patient to have optimal nursing care post procedure. Not knowing can lead to lapses in the level of patient care while the location and personnel are being sorted out.

INFECTION CONTROL

For the best practice, the procedural suites and the neuro-angiography suite should base their policy and procedure guidelines for infection control on the recommendations of the Association of periOperative Registered Nurses (AORN, 2012).

Fast Facts

Quality infection-control behavior protects both patients and healthcare workers by preventing transmitting microorganisms.

All personnel who enter the semirestricted and restricted areas of the angiography suite should wear surgical attire intended for use within the angiography suite. The procedural attire should be laundered within the institution.

Fast Facts

Remember: *It is all about the patient*!
For success in your practice, make your actions better than they "have" to be:
- Use evidence-based medicine and nursing.
- Pay attention to every detail.
- Recognize that "minimally invasive" procedures are still *invasive*.
- Run your angio suite like an operating room.

Personnel should cover head and facial hair, including sideburns and necklines, within the semirestricted and restricted areas of the angiography suite at all times. Hair can collect bacteria when left uncovered and potentially contribute to a wound infection. This makes it necessary for hair to be covered at all times. All personnel entering restricted areas of the angiography suite should wear a mask when sterile items and equipment are exposed. Masks are intended to contain and filter droplets containing microorganisms expelled from the mouth and nasopharynx during talking, sneezing, and coughing. Gloves should be selected and worn, depending on the task to be performed, as follows:

- Sterile gloves for sterile procedures.
- Unsterile gloves for other tasks including any encounter with body fluids or potentially infective material.
- Change gloves after each task and between patients to reduce the risk of spread of infection. Hand hygiene should be performed before and after donning all gloves (Spry, 1997).

Fast Facts

- Healthcare workers with artificial nails are more likely to carry pathogens than those with native nails.
- Artificial nails harbor more bacteria than with natural nails, even with scrubbing. https://www.cdc.gov/handhygiene/providers/index.html.
- Avoidance of artificial fingernails or extenders when providing patient care is a Category 1A recommendation, supported by well-designed experimental, clinical, or epidemiologic studies and strongly recommended.

Hand hygiene and proper use of appropriate barriers such as gowns, gloves, and masks help prevent avoidable infections by potentially drug-resistant pathogens. Everyone involved in the procedure should don a hat and mask prior to entering the procedure room. The patient should wear a surgical cap but does not need a mask on during the procedure. A surgical scrub should be done prior to setting up the sterile tray. Surgical scrub and sterile gown and gloves should be worn by the operator and scrub assistant. Do not have food in the procedure area: It risks attracting flies that can spread an infection to the procedure room. (It is also torture for a patient who may be fasting to smell food.)

Why Pay Attention to Infection Control

- Infections can adversely affect patient outcome.
- Mandates compliance with organizational infection-control policies.
- Infection control required by The Joint Commission Guidelines.
- Hospital-based infections are increasing.
- Hospital-based infections trigger penalties for insurance payments to hospitals.
- Implantation of devices can potentially increase the risk of infection.
- Increased use of closure devices, which involve implantation of a foreign body.
- Bacteremia can occur in 32% of angiography cases over 2 hours.
  - Drug-resistant "superbugs" are now everywhere.

Infection control protects patients and healthcare workers. Personal protective equipment (hats, masks, gloves, gowns, face shields) prevent infective material from patients contaminating the healthcare worker. The arteriogram is a prime example of a procedure in which a patient's blood may potentially spurt during puncture of the artery, spray as blood-contaminated wires or catheters are whipped around, and many other ways in which blood may be transferred to unprotected personnel. Routine hospital laundering of surgical scrubs and *never* wearing hospital scrubs anywhere outside the hospital will help prevent the spreading of all the infective material that may splash or spray during these procedures.

The Hallmarks of Universal Precautions

- Take precautions always, even if you do not suspect a dangerous infectious disease.
- Hats, masks, gloves, gown, and face shields should be worn when performing an invasive procedure.
- Wear gloves when handling body fluids.

Fast Facts

In 1999, New York State signed the following into law: Professionals who do not adhere to scientific infection-control policies are guilty of unprofessional conduct.

PATIENT SAFETY

The patient is someone we have been given the privilege and responsibility to treat and protect. Their life is in our hands. Working as a team allows one to ensure high-quality and safe care for our patients. Essential to patient safety are:

Patient Identification

Crucial prior to the start of any procedure, the "Time Out" procedure should include:

- Two patient identifiers (name, date of birth, medical record number).
- What procedure is to be done (verify procedural orders, specimen orders, etc.).
- Consents (procedural, sedation, blood, do not resuscitate [DNR] orders, etc.).
- Dry-erase board mounted on the wall for key information about the patient and the procedure will provide a quick visual for all members of the team.
- The procedure nurse is responsible for:
  - Reviewing the patient's neurological status.
  - Baseline vital signs, current lab work, medications, allergies, weight, and medical history.
  - Documents are in order (consents, electronic documents, and so on).

Hemodynamic Monitoring

Place all patients on hemodynamic monitoring on admission to the angiography suite and throughout procedure. Notify attending physician of any abnormalities.

Fast Facts

- All invasive transducers should be attached to the angiography table and zeroed as the table may be raised and lowered multiple times throughout the procedure.
- This prevents over-/under-draining of cerebral spinal fluid from the ventriculostomy (and prevents intracranial crisis).
- This maintains accurate measurements from arterial lines or central lines.

Medication Safety

- Drug allergies should be known prior to the procedure and listed on the dry-erase board in the procedure room.
- Patient weight in kilograms should be known and also written on the board.
- Follow organizational policy to ensure proper medication dosage.
  - Read labels carefully.
  - Always check and double-check doses.
  - Utilize a second nurse to confirm for critical medications, such as heparin.
- Refer to Chapter 7, Sedation and Monitoring, for more information on procedural sedation and monitoring.

Documentation Safety

- Routine documentation of vital signs, medications, and patient assessment should be precise throughout the procedural case.
- Documentation of implanted devices (coils, stents, closure devices, etc.) should include the lot number and expiration date.
  - This could have important implications for the patient's future (MRI compatibility, recall of implanted device, etc.).
- Refer to Chapter 8, Documentation, for more information on documentation in the radiology setting.

General Safety Tips

- Smaller is better (very important in pediatrics).
  - Use the smallest vascular access possible; this may be femoral or radial.
- Heparin is your friend.
  - Prevents thrombus on catheter.
- Label all containers on tray and all syringes (The Joint Commission requirement).
- Empty syringes on the sterile procedural table should *never* be full of air.
  - Either fill the syringes with heparinized saline or contrast.
- Air bubbles are *not* your friends during neuroangiography.
- Repetition is your friend.
- Items can only be either sterile or contaminated: There is no in-between!

- Eye shields should be worn by all personnel and by patient during glue embolization with Trufill Glue (Codman, Raynham, MA). *No way to undo effects of glue if splash occurs.*
- Angiographic procedures are truly team efforts.
  - Every team member is essential, and everyone has their area of expertise.
  - Everyone must perform at the top of their game.
  - Only when the whole team is patient-focused can the institution rise above the ordinary (Harrigan & Deveikis, 2018).

PATIENT EDUCATION ON NEUROINTERVENTIONAL PROCEDURES

Key topics to be thoroughly explained are as follows:

- Preprocedural:
  - Medication information, lab work, appointments, and so forth.
  - Patient should be allowed time to ask any and all questions they may have.
- Intraprocedural:
  - The patient must be made a team member who is actively involved with getting the procedure accomplished safely and effectively.
  - Coax the patient to cooperate during key portions of the procedure.
  - Patients need to be warned before they might feel anything uncomfortable or unexpected.
- Postprocedural:
  - Discuss admission expectations or homecare.
  - Advise the patient with what they should/should not do, and what symptoms to expect, such as:
    - It is generally recommended that patients drink plenty of fluids after angiographic procedures.
    - Patients who have had a closure device placed should not sit in a tub or go swimming for 5 days post procedure.
    - Most patients may experience some access site tenderness after the local anesthetic wears off, but severe or persistent pain could be a sign of problems like hematoma or infection.
- Follow-up appointments.
- Provide written instructions prior to discharge.
- Be prepared to answer follow-up phone calls if the patient has any questions or problems (Baker, 2008).

Unanticipated movement during aneurysm coil placement or during n-butyl cyanoacrylate (n-BCA) embolization can be very serious for the patient. Movement may cause the catheter or coil to perforate the aneurysm and degrade image during deposit of n-BCA. Either of these occurrences may lead to a life-threatening scenario.

PATIENT COMFORT

A professional and clean environment must be maintained at all times. The temperature in the room should be maintained for patient comfort. Blanket warmer/cooler may be used for optimal temperature regulation for longer cases. Angiography rooms are frequently cold for the comfort of operating personnel wearing hats, masks, gowns, gloves, and lead protection aprons. However, always remember that the patient may be too cold, which can affect their comfort and ability to remain motionless without shivering. It can even have hemodynamic effects on the patient.

Other Comfort Tips

- Patient's modesty and privacy should be maintained at all times.
- Support and reassurance should be provided to all patients.
- Excess noise, stimulation, and conversation should be kept to a minimum, especially during induction of anesthesia.
- Avoid distracting conversation: The patient should always be the central focus.
  - Laughing and joking heard in the room may make the patient feel uncomfortable and believe *they* are the subject of ridicule, even though it may be an unrelated conversation.
- Do not have food in the procedure area:
  - It is torture for a patient who may be fasting to smell food.
  - Risk of attracting insects.
  - Follow the AORN Guidelines.
- Arm and heel supports and padding should be used throughout the procedure to prevent possible ulna nerve and heel damage.
  - The patient's fingers should fit inside the arm supports at all times.
- Foley catheters should be placed if procedure is anticipated to be over 2 hours, with the patient asleep whenever possible for comfort and modesty.

- Secure the Foley with a little slack in the tubing to prevent inadvertent tension on the catheter.
- Foley bags should be hung on the side of the angiography table to decrease risk of infection from reflux into the bladder and to accurately measure output (Cammermeyer & Appeldorn, 2010).

Fast Facts

Staff should:

- Treat each patient as an individual
- Understand how their disease process and the procedure can impact them
- Pay close attention to every detail

Only when the whole team is patient focused can the institution rise above the ordinary.

CRISIS MANAGEMENT

The team should be prepared for the worst-case scenario for each procedure performed. Emergency crash cart and medication must be readily available. Be familiar with the equipment and know where important items are stored. Verify that every patient has two *functioning* IVs (preferably 18G or larger). They should be checked for patency prior to groin access. It can be difficult and time-consuming to place the second IV while the patient is crashing. Place all IV poles and anesthesia equipment out of the way of the x-ray equipment. Consider Advanced Cardiac Life Support (ACLS) certification if you are involved with angiographic procedures. This certification is also mandatory for many departments.

Have Readily Available

- Emergency crash cart
- Medications
- Oxygen
- Suction (make sure suction can reach the length of the angiography table)
- Appropriate-size Ambu bag
- Masks
- Equipment for intubation

- Point-of-care glucose testing capability, especially in diabetic patients who have a sudden change in neurological status
- An extra bag of saline in case you need to give volume in a hurry

Emergencies

Contrast Reaction

Check for history of allergies and premedicate patients with a history of contrast allergy. Be suspicious after contrast has been given when patient shows restlessness, itchiness, or an increased respiratory rate. This could be the first sign of an anaphylactic reaction. Be prepared to rapidly give oxygen or intravenous (IV) fluids and have rescue medications available. Refer to Chapter 12 for additional information on iodinated contrast reactions and treatment.

Aneurysm Rupture

Anticipate a decline in patient's neurological status. If patient is not intubated, this may need to be done emergently. If the patient becomes hemodynamically unstable, they may need to be supported with volume and blood pressure support. The affected vessel may need to be temporarily shut down with either a balloon or coils emergently. If the patient has a ventriculostomy (EVD) catheter in place, a rapid change in intracranial pressure (ICP) may indicate aneurysm rupture and it may be necessary to open the catheter to drain. Patients without a preexisting catheter may need an emergent ventriculostomy placed. Have necessary equipment and access to someone who can set up the system.

Carotid Angioplasty or Carotid Stenting Crisis

Especially if working with a de novo carotid (never had surgery), patient may develop severe bradycardia and hypotension. Have atropine available. Always have a pacer available and place pacer pads prior to start of procedure. Know how to operate the pacer. Carotid ruptures during angioplasty or stent placement may need to sacrifice the carotid or temporize bleeding with a balloon occlusion.

Groin Site Complications

Hematoma can be life-threatening and threaten the circulation in the affected limb resulting in amputation. Hematomas can occur even when closure devices are used. Monitoring of puncture site should be strictly adhered to. Sandbags are not recommended for hematoma because they give a false sense of security. The hematoma goes unrecognized until it expands past the circumference of the bag, allowing for greater expansion of the hematoma. Apply pressure dressing in cases when you might expect hematoma formation, such as older patients with friable vessels, on anticoagulation or very obese patients. Excessive groin or back pain should be investigated since pain can be the first sign of a retroperitoneal bleed or expanding hematoma in the leg. If you suspect active bleeding, you may need to puncture opposite groin to diagnose and possibly treat cause of bleeding. Always check the color, temperature, and distal pulses of the accessed limb to rule out an ischemic problem as well (Harrigan & Deveikis, 2018).

Fast Facts

Making the *perfect* pressure dressing:

- Cover pubic hair (comfort measure for removing dressing).
- Place about eight 4-by-4-inch gauze pads at puncture site.
- Apply Elastoplast (BSN Medical Inc., Charlotte, NC) over the 4-by-4-inch gauze, crossing from one iliac crest to the other iliac crest. Apply a second layer of Elastoplast crossing over the first layer.
- The pressure dressing should be supportive but should not cause discomfort.
- The pressure dressing should be left in place for no more than 12 hours.
- This can be very effective in controlling hematomas.
- Continue routine neurovascular checks of extremity.

References

Association of periOperative Registered Nurses. (2012, December). Recommended practices for prevention of transmissible infections in the perioperative setting. *Perioperative Standards and Recommended Practices*, e91–e123. doi:10.1016/j.aorn.2013.08.018

Barker, E. (2008). *Neuroscience nursing: A spectrum of care* (3rd ed.). St. Louis, MO: Mosby.

Cammermeyer, M., & Appeldorn, C. (Eds.). (2010). *Core curriculum for neuroscience nursing* (5th ed.). Chicago, IL: American Association of Neuroscience Nurses.

Harrigan, M. R., & Deveikis, J. P. (2018). *Handbook of cerebrovascular disease and neurointerventional technique* (3rd ed.). New York, NY: Springer Publishing Company.

Spry, C. (1997). *Essentials of perioperative nursing*. Gaithersburg, MD: Aspen.

16

Neurointerventional Procedures for Ischemia

Susan Deveikis and John P. Deveikis

The nervous system is vitally important for the normal functioning of the individual, yet the brain is very sensitive to ischemia. Acute ischemic stroke can have disabling effects on patients. This chapter covers neurointerventional procedures that are minimally invasive treatments for cerebral ischemia. These procedures can complement or sometimes replace more traditional medical and surgical treatments for these conditions. The subsequent chapter covers the neurointerventional embolization procedure.

In this chapter, you will discover:

1. Preprocedural, intraprocedural, and postprocedural basics
2. Anticipating and preparing for complications
3. Rapid stroke care by all team members for improved outcomes
4. The nurse's role in neurointerventional procedures

Exhibit 16.1

Preprocedural Workup Basics

- Elective patients seen in the preoperative clinic. Emergent patients seen in the ED or in the ICU.
- Provide nothing by mouth after midnight; get consent signed.
- Identification/consideration of the possibility that the patient is pregnant.
- Assess allergies, neurological status, medical history, recent imaging, current reviewed labs if available, and medications.
- Provide reassurance and education to patient and family throughout procedure.
- For outpatients, confirm designated driver prior to starting procedure.
- Have patient void if no Foley catheter.
- Remove all jewelry and secure per hospital policy.
- Obtain baseline vital signs and pedal pulses prior to groin puncture.
- Patent intravenous (IVs) (at least 18 g or 16 g), 0.9% normal saline.
- Antibiotics may be given.
- Have suction, Ambu bag, and emergency drugs readily available prior to patient's arrival.
- Anticipate post procedure bed status.

Exhibit 16.2

Intraprocedural Care Basics

- Verify patient identification upon arrival to angiography suite.
- Obtain baseline neurological status; monitor for any subtle change in neurological assessment.
- Never leave patient unattended. Provide emotional support to patient.
- Place patient on hemodynamic monitors and obtain baseline vital signs. Monitor and record throughout procedure unless performed by anesthesia team.
- Pad patient's elbows and heels (to prevent skin or nerve damage) and place patient's head in head sponge in a neutral position.
- Place sequential compression device on bilateral lower extremities.
- "Time out" prior to groin puncture or per institutional policy.
- If Foley catheter required: Place using sterile technique after induction of general anesthesia and prior to groin prep and drape.

Exhibit 16.2

Intraprocedural Care Basics (*continued*)

- Clip groin according to department's infection-control policy. May be done by technologist or circulator.
- Prep and drape in a sterile manner. Follow manufacturer's recommendations for drying time prior to draping patient.

Exhibit 16.3

Postprocedural Care Basics

- Obtain postprocedural pedal pulses, check groin puncture site upon completion of procedure and then every 15 minutes × 3, every 30 minutes × 2, and every 1 hour × 1.
- Strict bedrest with accessed leg extended for 1 to 2 hours if closure device placed (or 6 hours if no closure device used).
- If radial arterial access site, use balloon wrist band (TR band [radial artery compression device], Terumo, Somerset, NJ) and slowly deflate according to recommended protocol.
- Neurological exam upon completion of procedure and then per protocol.
- Call report to receiving nurse.
- Accompany patient to receiving department.
- Unless nothing by mouth (NPO), encourage oral fluids post procedure, 100 mL over next 4 hours.
- Resume preprocedure diet and medications as indicated (Barker, 2008; Spry, 1997).

NEURONTERVENTIONAL PROCEDURES FOR ISCHEMIA

Endovascular Ischemic Stroke Treatment

Description

Resolution of acute arterial or venous occlusion via catheterization and extraction of thrombus.

Indications

- New-onset neurological deficit caused by an acute cerebral thrombus, a large vessel occlusion that is accessible by the appropriate catheter systems.
- Current guidelines state selected patients may be candidates for endovascular treatment up to 24 hours from symptom onset.

Preprocedural Care

- Refer to Exhibit 16.1 for basic preprocedural care.
- Nothing by mouth—but usually done on an emergent basis.
- Consent usually signed by next of kin or an emergent consent obtained.
- Anticipate ICU post procedure.
- Assess time when patient was last seen normal, allergies, neurological status, The National Institutes of Health (NIH) stroke scale, medical history, recent imaging to exclude intracranial bleeding, current reviewed labs if available, medications such as tissue plasminogen activator (tPA) or anticoagulants.
- Emergency evaluation in the ED, ICU, or upon arrival at the angiography suite.
- Have protamine, heparin, tPA, nicardipine, and abciximab available at all times.

Anesthesia

- Anesthesia may or may not be used, operator preference.

Intraprocedural Care

- Refer to Exhibit 16.2 for basic intraprocedural care.
- Conduct frequent neurological assessments and communicate any changes to attending physician immediately.
- Anticipate worst-case scenario, such as cerebral edema or hemorrhage.
- Ensure point-of-care coagulation test (activated clotting time) capability.
- Prior to recanalization, blood pressure may need to be supported to maximize perfusion. After recanalization, blood pressure may need to be decreased to prevent reperfusion injury and hemorrhage.
- Emergent intubation may be necessary depending on patient's ability to protect their airway. Assist anesthesia during emergent intubation if necessary or line placement if necessary.
- If Foley catheter required, it should be placed using sterile technique, *but do not delay procedure to place Foley catheter.* Strongly recommended if patient is aphasic and hemiplegic. Encourage placement prior to tPA and endovascular procedure, if possible.
- Be familiar with the use of aspiration catheter and stent retrievers from various manufacturers (Penumbra, Stryker, Medtronic, Codman).

Fast Facts

- Acute stroke *must* be treated rapidly.
- Neurons are dying rapidly (*1.9 million/minute*), so any delay can worsen outcome.
- Do not waste time with tasks that can be done later (e.g., Foley catheter placement, talking about the next case).
- This is an *emergency*, and the entire team needs to focus on caring for the patient quickly.

Postprocedural Care

- Refer to Exhibit 16.3 for basic postprocedural care.
- Anticipate ICU post procedure.
- Continue NPO until after completion of swallow study.
- Monitor access site carefully especially if previously on anticoagulation therapy and/or tPA.

Follow-Up

- May perform immediate postprocedure CT if concerned for acute hemorrhage or otherwise routinely done within 24 hours.
- Workup for cause of stroke and preventing possible recurrence.

Carotid Stenting

Description

- Dilation of narrowed segment by inflating a balloon (angioplasty) followed by placement of cylinder mesh to maintain normal vessel caliber and increase blood flow to the brain.

Indication

- Symptomatic in spite of maximal medical therapy and not a good candidate for open surgical endarterectomy.

Preprocedural Care

- Refer to Exhibit 16.1 for basic preprocedural care.
- Anticipate ICU post procedure.
- Obtain assessments including allergies, neurological status, medical history, current reviewed labs.
- Provide patient education. Elective patients will be seen in the preoperative clinic prior to procedure. Emergency patient's evaluation will be done in the hospital.

- Antibiotics may be given prior to implantation of stent.
- Antiplatelet agents may be loaded immediately prior to procedure or may have been started several days before.
- Have heparin, protamine, atropine, and abciximab available at all times.

Anesthesia
- Usually done without anesthesia.

Fast Facts

- Inflation of a balloon at the carotid bifurcation can stimulate the pressure receptors in the vessel wall and result in sudden, often severe bradycardia and hypotension.
- Worst-case scenario: Patient may become asystolic.
- Mild cases may resolve as soon as balloon is deflated.
- Intravenous atropine may help with persistent bradycardia.
- Be prepared to administer external pacing for severe bradycardia with hypotension.

Intraprocedural Care
- Refer to Exhibit 16.2 for basic intraprocedural care.
- Place temporary pacer pads on patient prior to procedure; have temporary pacer in room during procedure.

Postprocedural Care
- Refer to Exhibit 16.3 for basic postprocedural care.
- Anticipate ICU post procedure. Possible reperfusion injury after stent placement.
- May perform postprocedure CT if clinical concern for hemorrhage.
- Resume preprocedure medications, including dual antiplatelet drugs.

Follow-Up
- Clinic 2 weeks post procedure.
- Ultrasound/duplex study within 2 weeks and 6 months post procedure (Harrigan & Deveikis, 2018).

Intracranial Angioplasty

Description

- Increase caliber of narrowed intracranial vessels using a balloon (angioplasty) and/or vasodilator for arteries narrowed by vasospasm from subarachnoid hemorrhage (SAH). Arteries narrowed due to atherosclerotic plaque are dilated using balloon angioplasty with or without stent implantation to maintain vessel patency.

Indications

- Decrease in neurological status or delayed new focal deficit following SAH or repeated neurological events from atherosclerotic stenosis in spite of maximal medical therapy.

Preprocedural Workup

- Refer to Exhibit 16.1 for basic preprocedural care.
- Anticipate continued ICU post procedure.
- Emergency patient's evaluation will be done in the ICU and upon arrival to the angiography suite.
- Have protamine, heparin, nicardipine, and abciximab available at all times.

Anesthesia

- Anesthesia usually required due to pain from intracranial balloon angioplasty.

Intraprocedural Care

- Refer to Exhibit 16.2 for basic intraprocedural care.
- Assist with anesthesia, if necessary; secure intracranial pressure monitor if in place.

Fast Facts

- The most-feared complication from intracranial angioplasty is vessel rupture.
- Always look for sudden change in vital signs or ICP, usually immediately after balloon inflation.
- Patients not under anesthesia always experience some transient discomfort during balloon inflation, but it would be more severe and persistent if the vessel ruptures (Cammermeyer & Appeldorn, 2010).

Postprocedural Care

- Refer to Exhibit 16.3 for basic postprocedural care.
- Continue ICU care post procedure and be vigilant for possible reperfusion injury post angioplasty.
- Maintain IV fluids running with 0.9% NaCl.

Follow-Up

- May do post procedure CT if clinical concern for new hemorrhage.
- Patient to be followed up in hospital and then seen in clinic 2 weeks post procedure or 2 weeks post hospitalization.
- After angioplasty for vasospasm, angiographic follow-up as per routine post-aneurysm therapy, usually in 6 months, then angiography or magnetic resonance angiography (MRA) annually.
- For angioplasty of atherosclerotic disease, angiography or computed tomographic angiography (CTA), follow-up in 3 to 6 months and long-term follow-up with either angiography or CTA annually.

Test Occlusion

Description

- Temporary occlusion of a vessel using a balloon to test for tolerance if that vessel must be occluded. Most commonly done in the internal carotid artery. The patient is tested neurologically during the test to evaluate for new neurological deficits, which would indicate that the patient would not tolerate permanent occlusion of that vessel. Often a cerebral blood flow test such as CT perfusion or nuclear medicine single photon emission computed tomography (SPECT) scans are done during the test occlusion to further evaluate what the occlusion would do to brain blood flow.

Indications

- Tumor or giant aneurysm involving the vessel, which may require permanent occlusion of the vessel to treat the lesion.

Preprocedural Care

- Refer to Exhibit 16.1 for basic preprocedural care.
- Coordinate with the OR the date and time of surgery, if planned.

- Coordinate the desired cerebral blood flow test that is to be done during the test.
- Obtain baseline neurological status.
- Anticipate floor bed after procedure; ICU usually not necessary.
- Antibiotics usually not given prior to procedure.

Anesthesia

- General anesthesia usually not used due to neurological testing.

Intraprocedural Care

- Refer to Exhibit 16.2 for basic intraprocedural care.
- Obtain baseline neurological status; monitor for any subtle change in neurological assessment throughout the procedure.
- If blood flow testing will be done, be prepared for transport to the CT scanner for CT perfusion or have the nuclear tracer available for nuclear SPECT imaging.
- Document results of neurological testing.

Fast Facts

- Decrease in level of consciousness or focal deficit may mean the patient cannot tolerate the occlusion.
- One trick is to give the patient a rubber squeaky toy in their hand contralateral to the vessel being occluded and have them squeeze it repeatedly during the balloon inflation.
- If the squeaking stops, the patient may be developing a hemiparesis.

Postprocedural Care

- Refer to Exhibit 16.3 for basic postprocedural care.
- Anticipate floor status post procedure if procedure is extracranial and no anticipation of post procedure deficits.

Follow-Up

- Patient is usually seen in the clinic 2 weeks post procedure.
- Imaging follow-up per surgeon.

Petrosal Venous Sampling

Description

- Patients with elevated cortisol levels may have a pituitary tumor that produces adreno-corticotropic hormone (ACTH). This is called Cushing's disease. Some of these tumors may be too small to localize on MRI scans. Sampling blood from the veins draining the pituitary may be done by catheterization and sampling from the inferior petrosal sinus. Measuring has a high accuracy of localizing the tumor in the pituitary gland, and often can determine which side of the gland is involved, allowing for surgical cure of the Cushing's disease. A stimulant of pituitary function (e.g., corticotropin releasing hormone [CRH] or 1-deamino-8-D-arginine vasopressin [DDAVP]) is often given during the test to increase accuracy.

Indications

- Symptoms and laboratory evidence of Cushing's disease without a clear-cut tumor explaining the abnormal hormone production.

Preprocedural Care

- Refer to Exhibit 16.1 for basic preprocedural care.
- Coordinate with the lab date and time of procedure. Be sure to know the proper tubes needed for the samples, and make sure the lab understands the large number of samples they will be receiving and how they will be labeled.
- Anticipate floor status post procedure or may be done as outpatient.
- Antibiotics usually not used.
- Have available heparin, protamine, CRH, or other pituitary stimulant.
- Have appropriate tubes for samples, labels, worksheet to document time, site and number of samples, and an ice bath to keep the samples when transported to the lab.
- Ensure that each member of the team knows what their role will be when the samples are taken.

Anesthesia

- General anesthesia is usually not used due to its effect on pituitary function. Sedatives can reduce the accuracy of the test.

Fast Facts

- Petrosal sinus sampling requires multiple catheters with simultaneous blood samples obtained from each of the right and left petrosal sinuses and a peripheral venous sample usually obtained from a femoral venous sheath.
- These samples are obtained at various time intervals before, and then repeated after the pituitary stimulating drug (e.g., CRH or DDAVP) is given.
- Samples are tested for ACTH levels.
- Simultaneous samples mean several operators are needed to obtain the samples; then several circulators must take the samples, put them in proper tubes, and label them carefully.
- There will be many samples with many opportunities for error.
- The results are only useful if one can be absolutely certain that they are correctly labeled as to whether it came from the right or left inferior petrosal sinus or peripheral vein *and* whether it was before or after pituitary stimulation.

Intraprocedural Care

- Refer to Exhibit 16.2 for basic intraprocedural care.

Postprocedural Care

- Refer to Exhibit 16.3 for basic postprocedural care.
- Anticipate floor status post procedure. May even be done as outpatient procedure.
- Strict bedrest with accessed legs extended for 1 hour if hemostatic patch placed or 2 to 3 hours if no hemostatic agent used.
- Head of bed elevated 20 degrees immediately post procedure to decrease risk of swelling.
- Ensure that properly labeled samples get to appropriate personnel in the lab.

Follow-Up

- Patient will be seen in the clinic 2 weeks post procedure.
- Imaging follow-up per surgeon.

Fast Facts

- Ischemic stroke and other cerebrovascular conditions can be devastating for the patient but can be treated with neurointerventional procedures.
- *Listen to your patient.* Always pay close attention to vital signs and neurological status. A sudden change can indicate something bad is happening.
- *Protect your patient.* Attention to detail with careful positioning of the patient, padding of extremities, and anticipating potential problems can keep the patient safe.
- *Talk to your patient.* Providing encouragement, support, and education can help them through the procedure.

References

Barker, E. (2008). *Neuroscience nursing: A spectrum of care* (3rd ed.). St. Louis, MO: Mosby.

Cammermeyer, M., & Appeldorn, C. (Eds.). (2010). *Core curriculum for neuroscience nursing* (5th ed.). Chicago, IL: American Association of Neuroscience Nurses.

Harrigan, M. R., & Deveikis, J. P. (2018). *Handbook of cerebrovascular disease and neurointerventional technique* (3rd ed.). New York, NY: Springer Publishing Company.

Spry, C. (1997). *Essentials of perioperative nursing.* Gaithersburg, MD: Aspen.

17

Neurointerventional Embolization

Susan Deveikis and John P. Deveikis

The nervous system is vitally important for the normal functioning of the individual, yet the brain is very sensitive to ischemia.
Disorders of the vascular supply to the nervous system can have devastating effects on patients and can be fatal. Neurointerventional
embolization procedures are minimally invasive treatments for
neurovascular conditions in which blood supply or an abnormal
vascular structure is blocked off or "embolized." These procedures
can complement or sometimes replace more traditional medical
and surgical treatments for these conditions.

In this chapter, you will discover:

1. Anticipating and preparing for complications
2. Meticulous attention to detail by all team members to ensure optimal outcomes
3. The nurse's role in neurointerventional embolization

NEUROINTERVENTIONAL EMBOLIZATION

Intracranial Aneurysm Embolization

Description

- Intracranial aneurysms can be treated by coil embolization
  ("coiling"), or other methods, using a small catheter

(microcatheter) navigated through the vascular system to deliver devices that prevent blood flow into the aneurysm and thereby prevent the aneurysm from bleeding.

- Historically, embolization was first developed to treat patients who could not be treated with open surgical techniques (craniotomy and clipping of the aneurysm). However, randomized studies have shown outcomes of patients treated with coil embolization compare very favorably to those treated by open clipping. Now, increasing numbers of patients with aneurysms are treated by embolization as the primary treatment.
- Most of the time, the aneurysm can be coiled without occluding the parent artery, since the coils remain stable in the aneurysm sac and do not block the artery. Sometimes, when there is a wide opening (neck) between the aneurysm and its parent artery, assisted coiling can be done, placing a stent or other bridging device in the artery over the aneurysm neck to prevent the coils from protruding into the artery and possibly blocking blood flow.
- Recently, special stent-like devices called flow-diverters have become available. These are deployed in the parent artery across the aneurysm neck. The stent is made of a fine meshwork of wires that can decrease flow to the aneurysm and cause it to clot off, even without the use of any coils in the aneurysm. Flow-diverters such as the Pipeline™ embolization device (Covidien, Irvine, CA) can be used for certain aneurysms, especially the large, wide-neck aneurysms of the carotid artery that can be difficult to treat with coil embolization.
- Other devices, such as the Woven Endo Bridge (WEB, Sequent Medical, Aliso Viejo, CA), are placed in the aneurysm sack and block flow at the aneurysm neck.
- Some aneurysms can only be treated by blocking both the parent artery as well as the aneurysm itself, but this may impair blood flow to the brain and cause a stroke, so this is only rarely done (Harrigan & Deveikis, 2018).

Indications

- Ruptured intracranial aneurysm with subarachnoid hemorrhage (SAH).
- Unruptured aneurysms.
- Size and configuration favorable to position coils in a stable fashion.
- Patient should not have contraindications for arterial access (e.g., severe atherosclerotic occlusions, active bacteremia).
- Especially if using a stent or flow-diverter, patient should not have contraindications for use of antiplatelet medications (aspirin and clopidogrel).

Preprocedural Care

- Refer to Exhibit 16.1 for basic preprocedural care.
- Anticipate ICU stay post procedure.
- Obtain physical assessment including allergies, neurological status, medical history, current labs (prothrombin time [PT], partial thromboplastin time [PTT], blood urea nitrogen [BUN], creatinine, chemistries, type and screen) and provide patient education. Elective patients will be seen in the preoperative clinic prior to procedure. Emergency patient's evaluation will be done in the ED or ICU.
- Antibiotics may be given prior to implantation of devices.
- Antiplatelet agents may be given prior to procedure or may have been loaded several days before. Consider testing for platelet aggregation prior to the procedure to determine the effectiveness of the antiplatelet regimen. Often patients may be resistant to the effects of clopidogrel.
- Have heparin, protamine, and abciximab (ReoPro® Merck & Co., Whitehouse Station, NJ) available at all times (Barker, 2008; Spry, 1997).

Anesthesia

- Evaluation per anesthesia personnel if anesthesia to be used.

Fast Facts

Protamine is contraindicated in:

- Patients who are hypersensitive or intolerant to protamine.
- Insulin-dependent diabetics (may experience life-threatening anaphylaxis).
- Vasectomized males.

Intraprocedural Care

- Refer to Exhibit 16.2 for basic intraprocedural care.
- Ongoing neurological assessment: Anticipate worst-case scenario of aneurysm rupture, rebleed, or ischemic stroke.
- If intracranial pressure (ICP) monitor is in place, be sure ICP is clamped prior to patient transfer to angiography table. Place patient on angiography table, secure, and rezero ICP.
- Assist with anesthesia during intubation or line placement, if necessary. Radial arterial line may be placed prior to induction or procedure.

- If Foley catheter is required, it should be placed after general anesthesia (for patient comfort) using sterile technique.
- Determine preferred access site (i.e., radial vs. femoral).
- Prep and drape in a sterile manner (Cammermeyer & Appeldorn, 2010)

Fast Facts

- Transducers for any pressure monitors such as arterial lines, central venous pressure, or ICP should always be attached directly to the angiography table.
- This is to ensure safety, prevent lines from being pulled, and receive accurate readings.
- Remember that the angiography table may be raised and lowered multiple times during the procedure.

Postprocedural Care

- Refer to Exhibit 16.3 for basic postprocedural care.
- Anticipate bed status prior to procedure. Elective patients will need ICU bed post procedure; ICU patient will continue in ICU post procedure.
- Neurological exam upon completion of procedure and per ICU protocol preferably every 1 hour × 24.

Fast Facts

- Always keep an eye on vital signs and ICP monitor: A sudden change can be the first sign of aneurysm rupture.
- Acute aneurysm during the procedure may require urgent placement of a ventriculostomy catheter to relieve pressure on the brain. Easy access to and familiarity with the ventricular catheter system can be life-saving.
- Any SAH patient not under anesthesia should be kept calm and in a quiet, dark, nonstimulating environment.

Follow-Up

- If elective coiling of unruptured aneurysm occurs, the patient may only be in the hospital for a day or two. Patient will be seen in follow-up clinic 2 weeks post procedure. Magnetic resonance angiography (MRA) should follow in 6 months, 12 months, and then annually.

- If patient had a SAH, the patient will be seen 2 weeks after hospital discharge. SAH patients may have a prolonged hospital stay to recover from the hemorrhage. Plan for an arteriogram in 6 months and then MRA in 12 months and then annually.

Intracranial Arteriovenous Malformation and Arterial Venous Fistula Embolization

Description

- Arteriovenous malformation (AVM) is a congenital abnormality resulting in a network (nidus) of connections between arteries and veins. Arterial venous fistula (AVF) is a direct connection between artery and vein, which can be congenital or acquired.

Indications

- Rupture or risk of rupture, focal neurological symptoms, seizures, hydrocephalus, cardiac failure.

Preprocedural Care

- Refer to Exhibit 16.1 for basic preprocedural care.
- Obtain physical assessments including allergies, neurological status, medical history, current reviewed labs, and current imaging and provide patient education. Elective patients will be seen in the preoperative clinic prior to procedure.
- Anticipate ICU post procedure.

Anesthesia

- General anesthesia usually necessary.

Intraprocedural Care

- Refer to Exhibit 16.2 for basic intraprocedural care.
- Assist patient onto the angiography table.
- Assist anesthesia during intubation or line placement if necessary. Radial arterial line may be placed prior to induction or procedure.
- If Foley catheter is required, it should be placed after general anesthesia for patient comfort using sterile technique.

Postprocedural Care

- Refer to Exhibit 16.3 for basic postprocedural care.
- Elective patients will need ICU bed post procedure; ICU patients will continue in ICU post procedure.
- Neurological exam upon completion of procedure and, per ICU protocol, preferably every (1) hour × 24.

Follow-Up

- Patient to be seen in clinic 2 weeks post procedure or 2 weeks post hospitalization.
- Adults need angiographic follow-up in 3 to 6 months.
- Children need angiographic follow-up in 3 to 6 months but need long-term follow-up with either CT or MRI every 2 to 3 years.

Intracranial Tumor Embolization

Description

- Neoplastic space-occupying lesion.

Indications

- Reduce tumor vascularity prior to surgery.
- Shrink symptomatic tumors in patients who are not candidates for surgery.

Preprocedural Work-Up

- Refer to Exhibit 16.1 for basic preprocedural care.
- Coordinate with the OR for date and time of surgery. Surgery should be done within 3 to 5 days of tumor embolization.
- Obtain history and physical assessments including allergies, neurological status, medical history, current reviewed labs, recent imaging. Provide patient education. Elective patients will be seen in the preoperative clinic prior to procedure.
- Obtain baseline vital signs and bilateral pedal pulses prior to groin puncture.
- Anticipate ICU post procedure due to potential swelling of tumor post embolization.

Anesthesia

- General anesthesia may or may not be used, depending on patient or physician preference.

Intraprocedural Care

- Refer to Exhibit 16.2 for basic intraprocedural care.
- Provocative testing is implemented to evaluate possible blood supply to nerve cell bodies or other dangerous anastomoses prior to embolization. Transient new deficits may occur after injecting an anesthetic agent in the vessel of interest.
- For provocative testing, have methohexital sodium (Brevital® JHP Pharmaceuticals, Parsippany, NJ), lidocaine 2% Cardiac Bristo Jet, and sodium bicarbonate (pediatric 0.5 mEq/mL).

- For cases using nBCA glue for embolization, have 5% dextrose available.
- Document results of provocative testing for each vessel embolized or evaluated.

Fast Facts

- Decrease in level of consciousness or severe headache may mean intracranial tumor bleeding or swelling and need for emergent intracranial surgery.
- Be prepared to obtain STAT head CT scan if bleeding is suspected.
- High-dose steroids and mannitol can sometimes control swelling prior to surgery.

Postprocedural Care

- Refer to Exhibit 16.3 for basic postprocedural care.
- Anticipate bed status prior to procedure. Elective patients will need ICU bed post procedure; ICU patients will continue in ICU post procedure.
- Head of bed (HOB) elevated at least 20 degrees immediately post procedure.
- Neurological exam upon completion of procedure and, per ICU protocol, preferably every (1) hour × 24.

Follow-Up

- Patient will be seen in the clinic 2 weeks post procedure.
- Imaging follow-up per surgeon.

Extracranial Head and Neck Embolization

Description

- Block blood supply or control bleeding from a vascular lesion.

Indications

- Preoperative or to stop uncontrolled or recurrent bleeding.

Preprocedural Care

- Refer to Exhibit 16.1 for basic preprocedural care.
- Coordinate with the OR for date and time of surgery. Surgery should ideally be done within 3 to 5 days of embolization, unless done on emergent basis.

- Obtain physical assessments including allergies, neurological status, medical history, current reviewed labs (PT, PTT, BUN, creatinine), recent imaging. Provide patient education. Elective patients will be seen in the preoperative clinic prior to procedure.
- Anticipate floor bed after procedure; ICU usually not necessary.

Anesthesia

- General anesthesia usually not used due to provocative testing.

Intraprocedural Care

- Refer to Exhibit 16.2 for basic intraprocedural care.
- Point-of-care testing (activated clotting time) capability.
- For provocative testing, have methohexital sodium for IA injection, lidocaine 2% Cardiac Bristo Jet, sodium bicarbonate (pediatric 0.5 mEq/mL), and 5% dextrose available.
- Document results of provocative testing for each vessel embolized or tested.

Fast Facts

Preservative-free sterile water or normal saline must be used when mixing drugs for intra-arterial use.

Postprocedural Care

- Refer to Exhibit 16.3 for basic postprocedural care.
- Anticipate floor status post procedure if procedure is extracranial and no anticipation of post procedure swelling that could affect airway.
- HOB elevated 20 degrees immediately post procedure to decrease risk of swelling.

Follow-Up

- Patient to be seen in clinic 2 weeks post procedure.
- Post imaging per surgeon.

Spinal Embolization

Description

- The spine and spinal cord may be involved with vascular malformations and tumors that can be treated by catheter-based endovascular techniques. The procedure may be done prior to surgical resection of the lesion or as the primary mode of treatment. The technique is similar to what is used in the head and neck, but the arterial supply to the spine often includes small branches arising directly from the aorta. Great care should be taken to avoid blocking blood flow to the spinal cord, so usually before embolizing any spinal vessel, provocative testing is performed by injecting short-acting anesthetic agents (e.g., amobarbital, methohexital) into the feeding artery and testing for a transient neurological deficit. If the patient does not exhibit a new deficit, it means that the vessel to be embolized does not have any significant connection to the cord blood supply and it should be safe to embolize it.

Indications

- Spinal AVF.
- Spinal AVMs.
- Vascular tumors of the spine.

Preprocedural Care

- Refer to Exhibit 16.1 for basic preprocedural care.
- Coordinate with the OR for date and time of surgery if procedure is being done preoperatively.
- Obtain history and physical assessments including allergies, neurological status, medical history, current reviewed labs, and recent imaging. Provide patient education. Elective patients will be seen in the preoperative clinic prior to procedure.
- Anticipate ICU post procedure if due to potential swelling post embolization.
- Always have heparin, protamine, dexamethasone, methohexital or amobarbital, and lidocaine.

Anesthesia

- General anesthesia may or may not be used due to the use of provocative testing. Provocative testing is implemented to evaluate possible blood supply to nerve cell bodies or other dangerous anastomoses prior to embolization.
- Provocative testing in patients receiving general anesthesia is still possible if neurophysiological monitoring such as somatosensory or motor-evoked potentials is used. This monitoring must usually be scheduled well in advance of the procedure.

Intraprocedural Care

- Refer to Exhibit 16.2 for basic intraprocedural care.
- Frequent neurological assessment; communicate any changes to attending physician immediately.
- Point-of-care coagulation test (ACT) capability.

Postprocedural Care

- Refer to Exhibit 16.3 for basic postprocedural care.
- Anticipate floor status post procedure if procedure is extracranial and not directly involving spinal cord.
- HOB elevated 20 degrees immediately post procedure for comfort.

Follow-Up

- Patient will be seen in the clinic 2 weeks post procedure.
- Imaging follow-up per surgeon.

Fast Facts

- Ischemic stroke, subarachnoid hemorrhage, and other cerebrovascular conditions can be devastating for the patient but can be treated with neurointerventional procedures.
- *Listen to your patient.* Always pay close attention to vital signs and neurological status. A sudden change can indicate something untoward is happening.
- *Protect your patient.* Attention to detail with careful positioning of the patient, padding of extremities, and anticipating potential problems can keep the patient safe.
- *Talk to your patient.* Providing encouragement, support, and education can help them through the procedure.

References

Barker, E. (2008). *Neuroscience nursing: A spectrum of care* (3rd ed.). St. Louis, MO: Mosby.

Cammermeyer, M., & Appeldorn, C. (Eds.). (2010). *Core curriculum for neuroscience nursing* (5th ed.). Chicago, IL: American Association of Neuroscience Nurses.

Harrigan, M. R., & Deveikis, J. P. (2018). *Handbook of cerebrovascular disease and neurointerventional technique* (3rd ed.). New York, NY: Springer Publishing Company.

Spry, C. (1997). *Essentials of perioperative nursing.* Gaithersburg, MD: Aspen.

18

Basic (Body) Interventional Radiology Principles

Nana Ohene Baah and Ashwani Kumar Sharma

Caring for patients undergoing interventional radiology (IR) procedures requires a team of highly skilled procedural radiologists, radiologic technologists, nurses, and possibly anesthesiologists. Procedures performed will differ depending on the facility and the team: Some procedures are quite common and of a lower risk while other procedures carry a high risk and may mean life or death for a patient. Basic understanding is essential for all members of this team.

In this chapter, you will discover:

1. The importance of a sterile field and aseptic technique
2. Preprocedural/prophylactic antibiotic use
3. Pertinent lab values and preprocedural patient checklist

STERILE FIELD AND ASEPTIC TECHNIQUE

Sterile technique reduces the rate of procedure-related infections. Procedure-related bloodstream infections, including infections of prostheses and implanted devices, contribute significantly to patient morbidity and mortality. To protect the patient and the staff, adhere to strict aseptic technique at all times:

- Proper aseptic hand scrubbing before every procedure. Chlorhexidine gluconate- and ethyl alcohol-based scrubs and wipes provide the best protection against antimicrobial-resistant blood-borne pathogens.
- Disposable gowns, head cap, mask, and gloves required for each procedure.
- Care must be taken while draping the patient. Pay special attention to portable parts of the equipment table and other mobile equipment (e.g., ultrasound equipment, laser wand) that may require special drapes.
- The procedure site should be prepped while adhering to strict aseptic techniques.
- Patient's hair should be clipped at the site of the procedure using a disposable sterile clipper and hair shavings removed. The skin should be thoroughly prepped with chlorhexidine gluconate- and ethyl alcohol-based preparation for at least 2 minutes and allowed to dry. Alternatively, povidone–iodine can be used if patient has an allergy to chlorhexidine.
- All sterile packages used for the procedure should be checked for package integrity and expiration dates when applicable.
- Prior to commencement of the procedure, it is imperative that a *preprocedure "Time Out"* is performed by the attending physician after the patient is fully draped.

Fast Facts

Sterile technique and frequent handwashing are crucial for reducing the rate of infections in all IR procedures as well as improving patient care. Further information on sterile technique can be found at the U.S. Department of Health and Human Services at www.guideline.gov/content.aspx?id=12921#Section420.

ANTIBIOTICS

Prophylactic antibiotics can be given prior to IR procedures to reduce the chance of surgical site infection. Timing for intravenous (IV) antimicrobial prophylaxis should be as follows:

- Administered within 1 hour before and/or up to 3 hours after the procedure.

- Two hours prior to a procedure are allowed for the administration of vancomycin and fluoroquinolones.
- Intravenous antibiotics are usually given when the patient arrives to the angiography suite.

Choose the antibiotic based on the procedure:

- In *aseptic vascular procedures,* such as central venous catheter placement, a first-generation cephalosporin such as 1g of cefazolin IV is commonly used; alternatively, vancomycin can be used in a patient with penicillin or cephalosporin allergies.
- *Gram-negative bacterial* coverage in genitourinary interventions, such as percutaneous *nephrostomy* tube placement, is desired, and ciprofloxacin 400 mg IV can provide adequate prophylaxis.
- *Biliary interventions,* such as percutaneous biliary drains, require both gram-positive and gram-negative antibiotics with extended coverage. The dose of 3.375 g of IV Zosyn (piperacillin and tazobactam combination) is typically administered.

Table 18.1

Prophylactic Procedural Antibiotic Recommendations

Procedures	Routine Prophylaxis Recommendation	First Choice of Antibiotics	Alternative Antibiotics for Patients With Penicillin Allergy
Angiography Angioplasty Thrombolysis Arterial closure device placement Stent placement	No	Cefazolin in patients with risk for stent infection	Vancomycin or clindamycin
Biliary/liver procedures	Yes	No consensus; some may use ceftriaxone, Unasyn, or Zosyn	Vancomycin or clindamycin
Embolization and chemoembolization	Yes	No consensus; some may use ceftriaxone, cefazolin, and metronidazole, Unasyn, or Zosyn	Vancomycin
Gastrostomy	Yes for pull technique	Cefazolin	Vancomycin or clindamycin

(continued)

Table 18.1

Prophylactic Procedural Antibiotic Recommendations (*continued*)

Procedures	Routine Prophylaxis Recommendation	First Choice of Antibiotics	Alternative Antibiotics for Patients With Penicillin Allergy
GU procedures (include nephrostomy tubes and ureteral stents)	Yes (except for routine change in uninfected patients)	No consensus; some may use ceftriaxone, cefazolin, Unasyn or ampicillin and gentamicin	Vancomycin or clindamycin and Aminoglycoside
Percutaneous abscess drainage	Yes	No consensus; some may use ceftriaxone, cefoxitin, cefotetan, or Unasyn	Vancomycin or clindamycin or Aminoglycoside
Nephrostomy tubes	Yes	Ciprofloxacin	Vancomycin or clindamycin and aminoglycoside
Percutaneous biopsy (transrectal)	Yes	Gentamicin plus ciprofloxacin	
TIPSS creation	Yes	No consensus; some may use ceftriaxone, Unasyn, or Zosyn	Vancomycin or clindamycin and aminoglycoside
Tunneled central venous access	No consensus	Cefazolin in patients with history of catheter infection or immunosuppression	Vancomycin or clindamycin
Tumor ablation	No consensus	Some may use ceftriaxone, cefazolin, or Unasyn	Vancomycin or clindamycin
Uterine artery embolization	Yes	No consensus; some may use cefazolin, clindamycin and gentamycin or Unasyn	Vancomycin or clindamycin
Vertebroplasty	Yes	Cefazolin	Vancomycin or clindamycin

TIPSS, transjugular intrahepatic portosystemic shunt.

Source: Data from Chehab, M., Thakor, A. S., Tulin-Silver, S., Connolly, B. L., Cahill, A. M., Ward, T. J., & Venkatesan, A. M. (2018). Adult and pediatric antibiotic prophylaxis during vascular and IR procedures: A society of interventional radiology practice parameter update endorsed by the Cardiovascular and Interventional Radiological Society of Europe and the Canadian Association for Interventional Radiology. *Journal of Vascular and Interventional Radiology, 29*(11), 1483–1501.e2. doi:10.1016/j.jvir.2018.06.007

- Some of these antibiotics may require dose adjustment in patients with renal insufficiency.
- Refer to Table 18.1 for prophylactic procedural antibiotic guidelines during IR procedures.

COAGULATION STATUS AND HOMEOSTASIS

Procedures performed in IR often entail the puncturing of blood vessels or causing damage to visceral organs such as the kidney or liver. These procedures usually carry the risk of bleeding and/or hematoma at the access site. Therefore, screen patients for their bleeding risk and the ability to maintain homeostasis during and/or after the procedure.

Fast Facts

In emergent situations or in certain unique clinical scenarios, an interventional procedure will be performed if the benefits of the procedure outweigh the bleeding risk.

Several tests are used to assess the bleeding risk in patients; these include:

- Prothrombin time (PT)
  - Measure the extrinsic coagulation pathway
- International normalized ratio (INR)
  - Measure of the extrinsic coagulation pathway
  - Result is standardized and more dependable
  - Normal range is 0.9–1.1
- Activated partial thromboplastin time (aPTT)
  - Measure of the intrinsic coagulation pathway
  - Normal range for aPTT is 25 to 35 seconds
  - Patients receiving heparin or who have hemophilia may have an aPTT value of more than 50 seconds
- Platelet count
  - Normal platelet count is from 150,000 to 450,000 per microliter

Liver disease, vitamin deficiency, and oral anticoagulation therapy such as Coumadin (warfarin) can impair coagulation, resulting in a prolonged PT and elevated INR. The target INR for patients on Coumadin therapy is usually an INR of 2 to 3.5. Patients on anticoagulation therapy or who may have liver disease should have an INR/PT and platelets checked prior to IR procedures. Patients on heparin drips should have heparin drip discontinued 1 to 2 hours prior to the procedure or an aPTT can be checked.

The Journal of Vascular and Interventional Radiology consensus guidelines divide procedures into different categories depending on the risk of bleeding associated with the procedure.

Low Bleeding Risk Category

- Venography
- Arteriography (<6 French sheath)
- Inferior vena cava (IVC) filter placement
- Thoracentesis
- Paracentesis
- Chest tube placement
- Drainage catheter exchanges
- Dialysis access interventions
- Tunneled central line placement and removal

Routine testing of aPTT and INR is recommended for these low-risk procedures. For patients with risk factors, the target INR should be between 2 and 3, and platelets below 20,000 per microliter should be transfused.

High Bleeding Risk Category

- TIPSS
- Solid organ biopsies
- Ablations
- Arteriograms (>7 French sheath)
- Catheter-directed thrombolysis (deep vein thrombosis [DVT], pulmonary embolism [PE], portal vein)
- Biliary interventions
- Urinary tract interventions (nephrostomy tube placement, ureteral dilatation, stone removal)
- Venous interventions

Routine testing of platelets and INR is recommended for these high-risk procedures, with recommended thresholds for INR being less than 1.5 to 1.8. Platelet counts less than 50,000 per microliter should be transfused (see Table 18.2).

Plavix (Clopidogrel) should be held for 5 days prior to any high-risk-of-bleeding IR procedures. This sometimes requires consultation with the patient's cardiologist to ensure safety of the patient

Table 18.2

Coagulation Evaluation for Interventional Procedures		
Bleeding Risk	**Procedure**	**Recommendations**
Low bleeding risk	Dialysis access interventions	Lab screening for patients with risk factors:
	Venography	INR <2–3
	Central line removal	Platelets >20,000/ ul
	IVC filter placement	Not necessary to withhold clopidogrel, Prasugrel, Ticagrelor, UFH, low-molecular-weight heparin (LMWH), aspirin, short/long-acting nonsteroidal anti-inflammatory drugs (NSAIDs)
	PICC placement	
	Drainage catheter exchange	
	Thoracentesis	
	Paracentesis	
	Superficial aspiration; superficial soft tissue biopsy (e.g., thyroid biopsy)	
	Superficial abscess drainage	
	Angiography (<6 French sheath)	
	Venous interventions	
	Tunneled central venous catheter	
	Subcutaneous port device	
High bleeding risk	Arterial interventions (>7 French sheath)	Lab screening for patients with risk factors:
	Percutaneous ablations	INR ≤ 1.5–1.8
	Percutaneous cholecystostomy	Platelets >50,000/ul
	Intraabdominal, chest wall or retroperitoneal abscess drainage or biopsy	Withhold Clopidogrel, Ticagrelor 3–5days
	Solid organ biopsies (kidneys, liver, lung, adrenals)	Withhold 4–6 hr UFH Withhold 1 dose prophylactic and 2 therapeutic doses for LMWH
	Gastrostomy tube initial placement	

(continued)

Table 18.2

Coagulation Evaluation for Interventional Procedures (*continued*)		
Bleeding Risk	**Procedure**	**Recommendations**
	Spine procedures (vertebroplasty, kyphoplasty)	Check anti-factor Xa if impaired renal function; LMWH, aspirin, short/long-acting NSAIDs
	transjugular intrahepatic portosystemic shunt (TIPSS)	
	Renal biopsy	
	Percutaneous transhepatic cholangiogram (PTC)	
	Biliary drain initial placement	
	Nephrostomy tube initial placement	
	Radiofrequency ablation	

Source: Data from Patel, I. J., Rahim, S., Davidson, J. C., Hanks, S. E., Tam, A. L., Walker, T. G., & Weinberg, I. (2019). Society of interventional radiology consensus guidelines for the periprocedural management of thrombotic and bleeding risk in patients undergoing percutaneous image-guided interventions—Part II: Recommendations. *Journal of Vascular and Interventional Radiology, 30*(8), 1168–1184.e1. doi:10.1016/j.jvir.2019.04.017

while Plavix is being held. *Aspirin 325 mg or higher* should be held for 3 to 5 days prior to procedures with significant bleeding risks. Routine withholding is not recommended for low-risk procedures.

Low-molecular-weight *heparin* or *Lovenox* therapeutic doses should be held for 24 hours prior to the procedure (2 doses withheld), while IV heparin drip should be held for 4 to 6 hours prior to the procedure as heparin has a half-life of approximately one and half hours. Prophylactic doses of LMWH should be held for 12 hours (1 dose withheld).

Correction of coagulopathy may be necessary in patients requiring a procedure when the INR level or platelet counts do not meet the required recommendations.

Fresh frozen plasma (FFP) contains plasma proteins including coagulation factors and can be administered to patients with elevated INR.

Fast Facts

A platelet count >50,000/mL and an INR >1.5–1.8 are recommended to minimize the risk of excessive peri- and postprocedural bleeding in high-risk bleeding procedures.
Two units of FFP are usually sufficient to correct an INR of 2.5.

- When a procedure is emergently required for a patient with an elevated aPTT from a heparin drip and the procedure cannot be delayed, reversal medication protamine sulfate can be administered. Protamine dose is 1 mg per 100 units of heparin and has a rapid onset of 10 minutes; however, it has a short half-life of 5 to 7.5 minutes and repeat administration of protamine may be necessary.
- Patient with thrombocytopenia below the recommended platelet counts should receive transfusion with platelets prior to the procedure. Four to six units of random platelets or one unit of pooled platelets are frequently ordered. This transfusion can raise the platelet count by an estimated 30,000/ul.

MANAGEMENT OF CRITICALLY ILL PATIENTS

Critically ill patients are sometimes referred to IR for life-saving treatment. IR staff must be familiar with the basics of assessment and life-support management. Such cases include patients suffering from traumatic injury, patients with hemorrhage, and patients with severe disease such as liver failure or sepsis. Continuous monitoring of these patients to identify life-threatening problems during a procedure must be routinely performed. Observe the breathing rate and oxygen saturation during the procedure, and alert the physician for abnormal values.

Hypoxia

Hypoxia and hypoventilation during a procedure can be caused by many different reasons, including pneumothorax due to traumatic or iatrogenic injury, lung collapse due to mucus plugging, pulmonary edema or pleural effusion due to underlying systemic disease, and decreased respiratory drive due to sedation. When patients are hypoxic (pulse oximetry of less than 88–92%), consider applying or increasing supplemental oxygen with nasal cannula or high-flow oxygen mask, as well as identifying and acutely managing the underlying cause. Administration of reversal agents may be necessary if patients are reacting adversely to IV sedatives. Intubation may be required if patient is in respiratory failure.

Circulatory Compromise

Circulatory compromise during a procedure can be caused by many different reasons, including hemorrhage due to traumatic injury or gastrointestinal bleeding. Recognize that patients with:

- Hemorrhagic Class 1 (up to 15% loss of blood volume) have no significant change in vital signs.
- Hemorrhagic Class 2 (a blood loss of up to 30% of blood volume) features the early significant change of tachycardia and tachypnea.
- Hemorrhagic Class 3 (30–40% blood volume loss) results in oliguria, restlessness, and changes in skin perfusion.
- Hemorrhagic in Class 4 (>40% blood volume loss) results in hypotension, heart rate >140 bpm, and lethargy.
  - Adequate volume resuscitation is necessary when patients have signs of volume loss.
  - Initiate volume resuscitation with crystalloid IV fluids such as normal saline or lactated Ringer's solution.
  - Patients with hemorrhage may remain hypovolemic and after 1 to 2 L of crystalloid IV fluid may require packed red blood cell (PRBC) transfusions.
  - After four to six units of PRBCs are transfused, other blood products such as FFP, platelet, and cryoprecipitate can be considered.

Fast Facts

Patients with a left ventricular assist device (LVAD) may have a baseline of a lower automated blood pressure cuff measurement than non-LVAD patients. It could be as low as a systolic of 90 mmHg and be considered normal for that patient (Nassif et al., 2015). Manual cuff pressure with Doppler may be of benefit.

ANESTHESIA

Appropriate choice of medications in the management of pre- and periprocedural anxiety and discomfort helps patients undergo a technically and clinically successful procedure. Options for analgesia and anesthesia include local anesthesia, local anesthesia with sedation (mild, moderate, or deep), regional anesthesia, and general anesthesia. Local anesthesia with mild or moderate sedation is most commonly employed in IR procedures.

- Local anesthesia is achieved via infiltration of the skin with an amide such as lidocaine (1–3% concentrations are available as needed). In patients with a proven allergy to amides, esters such as procaine (available in 1% concentrations) have been safely used without any evidence of cross-reactive sensitivity.
- Mild sedation can be achieved by administering an IV dose of either a benzodiazepine or an opioid medication. When used in combination, the synergistic sedative effect provides moderate sedation (refer to Chapter 7, Sedation and Monitoring, for more information).
- Reversal agents such as flumazenil and naloxone should be readily available.
- Patient should maintain nothing by mouth (NPO) prior to the procedure per institutional policy. Typically, this includes no food or nonclear liquids for 6 to 8 hours and no clear liquids for 2 hours prior to administration of moderate sedation.
- Blood pressure, EKG, pulse oximetry, capnography, respiratory rate, and temperature should be monitored during procedures with sedation; vital signs should be recorded every 5 to 15 minutes per organizational policy. Supplemental oxygen with nasal cannula can be utilized to maintain patient's oxygenation.
- Postprocedure monitoring of patients for 30 minutes after the administration of the last dose of sedation is required.
- Some procedures can be performed with minimal sedation and only local anesthesia utilizing 1% lidocaine. Intraoperative monitoring for these procedures can be limited to blood pressure and EKG monitoring.

General anesthesia or deep sedation performed by the anesthesiology service is indicated in cases where patients are unable to tolerate the procedure with moderate sedation and local anesthesia. For instance, critically ill ASA Class III or IV patients (refer to Chapter 7, Sedation and Monitoring) who have difficulty maintaining their airway, patients with extreme anxiety that is poorly controlled with moderate sedation, and intellectually challenged patients may commonly undergo deep sedation or general anesthesia preprocedure. In pediatric cases, a pediatric intensivist or anesthesiologist typically provides sedation.

References

Chehab, M., Thakor, A. S., Tulin-Silver, S., Connolly, B. L., Cahill, A. M., Ward, T. J., & Venkatesan, A. M. (2018). Adult and pediatric antibiotic prophylaxis during vascular and IR procedures: A society of interventional radiology practice parameter update endorsed by the Cardiovascular and Interventional Radiological Society of Europe and the Canadian Association for Interventional Radiology. *Journal of Vascular and Interventional Radiology, 29*(11), 1483–1501.e2. doi:10.1016/j.jvir.2018.06.007

Nassif, M., Tibrewala, A., Raymer, D., Andruska, A., Novak, E., Vader, J., & LaRue, S. (2015). Systolic blood pressure on discharge after left ventricular device insertion is associated with subsequent stroke. *The Journal of Heart and Lung Transplantation, 34*(4), 503–508. doi:10.1016/j.healun.2014.09.042

Patel, I. J., Rahim, S., Davidson, J. C., Hanks, S. E., Tam, A. L., Walker, T. G., & Weinberg, I. (2019). Society of interventional radiology consensus guidelines for the periprocedural management of thrombotic and bleeding risk in patients undergoing percutaneous image-guided interventions—Part II: Recommendations. *Journal of Vascular and Interventional Radiology, 30*(8), 1168–1184.e1. doi:10.1016/j.jvir.2019.04.017

19

Interventions for Varicose Veins

*Nana Ohene Baah and
Ashwani Kumar Sharma*

Varicose veins are dilated, tortuous, and elongated veins that can affect up to 56% of men and 73% of women. Patients with varicose veins may complain of cosmetic deformity, pruritus, pain, swelling, cramping, or heaviness. Complications of varicose veins include thrombophlebitis, varicose eczema, lipodermatosclerosis, ulceration, and venous thrombosis.

In this chapter, you will discover:

1. Description of varicose veins
2. The different treatments available for varicose veins
3. Patient care through procedural phases

Exhibit 19.1

Preprocedural Care

- Provide nothing by mouth after midnight.
- Identify/consider pregnant/nonpregnant state.
- Remove all jewelry and secure per organizational policy.
- Have patient void prior to procedure.

(continued)

Exhibit 19.1

Preprocedural Care (*continued*)

- For outpatients, designated driver should be present prior to procedure.
- Verify medical history, including allergies and pregnancy, and check if physical assessments, including vital signs and appropriate lab results, are up to date.
- Obtain signature on consent forms (procedural, sedation, blood, do not resuscitate [DNR], etc.).
- Obtain baseline vital signs (including lung sounds, pedal pulses, etc., as appropriate).
- Place peripheral intravenous line(s).
- Anticipate postprocedural bed status.
- Check distal pulses before and after angiograms.

Exhibit 19.2

Intraprocedural Care

- Verify patient identification upon arrival to angiography suite.
- Check with operator for patient positioning.
- Never leave patient unattended. Provide emotional support to patient.
- Place patient on hemodynamic monitors (EKG, heart rate, blood pressure, respiratory rate, oxygen saturation, and capnography) and document baseline vital signs.
- Monitor and record throughout procedure per organizational policy.
- Ultrasound, fluoroscopy, or CT may be used depending on the case.
- Access site as determined by the physician.
- Hair at the site should be clipped, and the residue should be removed with tape (when appropriate).
- Prep and drape in a sterile manner (follow manufacturer's recommendations for drying time of skin prep prior to draping patient).
- "Time Out" and procedural verification prior to start of procedure should be per organizational policy.
- Samples obtained during a procedure require adequate labeling and handling per organizational policy.

Exhibit 19.3

Postprocedural Care

- Monitor patients in the postprocedure recovery area per organizational policy.
- Check access/puncture site for bleeding upon completion of the procedure and then hourly for signs of complications.
- Check distal pulses before and after angiograms.
- Resume preprocedure diet and medications as indicated.
- For outpatients, discharge instructions with contact information should be provided. Advise patient to seek medical attention if having swelling at procedure site, fevers, chills, or signs of allergic reaction.

VARICOSE VEINS

Varicose veins are dilated, tortuous, and elongated veins that can affect both males and females. Some studies suggest a prevalence of up to 56% in men and 73% in women. Patients with varicose veins may complain of cosmetic deformity, pruritus, pain, swelling, cramping, or heaviness. Complications of varicose veins include thrombophlebitis, varicose eczema, lipodermatosclerosis, ulceration, and venous thrombosis.

The veins of the lower extremity are divided into three categories: superficial, perforating, and deep veins. Superficial veins drain blood from the skin and subcutaneous tissues, act as a large reservoir, and drain periodically into larger superficial veins or into the deep venous system via the perforating veins. Normally, flow should be in the cephalad direction, and drain from the superficial to deep venous system. The deep veins are located deep in the muscle fascia in the legs and drain blood from muscles and blood that they receive from the superficial venous system via the perforating veins. The greater saphenous vein (GSV) is the largest of the superficial veins. The lesser saphenous vein (LSV) is the second truncal superficial vein.

Imaging studies are generally not necessary for diagnosis but are important for workup prior to planning treatment procedures. Evaluation of varicose veins is primarily assessed by duplex ultrasound examination (Wang & Sharma, 2019).

Fast Facts

The physical examination for the superficial veins is performed with the patient standing as that increases sensitivity and specificity.

Ablation for Varicose Vein

Introduction

- Endovenous laser ablation (EVLA) and radiofrequency ablation (RFA) are used to treat varicose veins that result from reflux in the greater saphenous and lesser saphenous veins. These work by inducing a thermal injury to the vein, which causes eventual fibrosis of the vein.
- Puncture is made into the vein of interest, and a vascular sheath is advanced into the vein. A laser sheath with a catheter or radiofrequency probe is then positioned appropriately under ultrasound or fluoroscopic guidance to perform the ablation.

Indications

- Symptomatic varicose veins with reflux in the greater or lesser saphenous and nonsaphenous veins
- Venous ulcers
- Varicose vein bleeding

Contraindications

- Deep venous thrombosis (DVT)
- Pregnancy
- Moderate-to-severe peripheral disease
- Joint disease that interferes with mobility

Preprocedural Care

- Refer to Exhibit 19.1 for basic preprocedural care.

Anesthesia

- Procedure is usually performed with perivenous tumescent anesthesia. Perivenous tumescent anesthesia is achieved by injecting a local anesthetic such as lidocaine around the vein targeted for therapy. Moderate sedation can also be given depending on the patient.

Intraprocedural Care

- Refer to Exhibit 19.2 for basic intraprocedural care.
- Patient is placed on a fluoroscopy table, usually in the supine position for saphenous vein and prone for lesser saphenous vein ablation.
- The procedure is performed with ultrasound and/or fluoroscopy.

Postprocedural Care

- Refer to Exhibit 19.3 for basic postprocedural care.

- Check site for bleeding or hematoma.
- Pain control is with acetaminophen or codeine. Nonsteroidal anti-inflammatory drugs (NSAIDs) should be *avoided* as these medications inhibit the inflammatory process, which is part of the goal of therapy to treat the varicose veins.

Complications

- Skin burn
- Nerve injury
- Superficial thrombophlebitis:
  - Superficial thrombophlebitis is a complication that is self-limited, peaks at 4 to 7 days, and resolves in approximately a week. Treatment includes ice packing. NSAIDs can be used cautiously for pain management and anti-inflammatory effect.

Follow-Up/Patient Education

- Follow up with interventional radiology 1 week post procedure.
- Ultrasound is used to evaluate for DVT in 1 week. The most concerning complication following endovenous laser ablation therapy is the development of a DVT, occurring in up to 5% of patients. It is for this reason that a follow-up ultrasound examination is performed approximately 1 week after the procedure.
- Patient should ambulate for 15 to 20 minutes several times a day.
- Compression stockings should be worn for 1 to 3 weeks post procedure. Patient may develop numbness in the lower extremities due to compression stockings; this can require removal of stockings and/or using lower pressure stockings.
- Avoid heavy lifting and strenuous activities for 1 to 2 weeks. Patient can usually return to normal activities in 3 to 7 weeks.
- Discharge instructions should advise patient to seek medical attention if having swelling at puncture site, swelling of the extremity, or severe pain suggesting DVT.

Phlebectomy for Varicose Vein

Introduction

- Phlebectomy is an ambulatory procedure that involves removal of varicose veins.
- Skin incisions as small as 1 to 3 mm or needle punctures using a needle are used to extract veins with a phlebectomy hook.

Indications

- Symptomatic varicose veins that are tortuous.

- Same indication for ablation but in cases that cannot be treated by ablation.

Contraindications

- Reflux at the saphenofemoral or saphenopopliteal junctions, which should be treated first before phlebectomy.

Preprocedural Care

- Refer to Exhibit 19.1 for basic preprocedural care.

Anesthesia

- Procedure usually performed with perivenous tumescent anesthesia as previously described.

Intraprocedural Care

- Refer to Exhibit 19.2 for basic intraprocedural care.
- Patient placed on fluoroscopy table, usually in supine position.
- Ultrasound or vein light is utilized.
- After allowing for drainage of anesthesia fluid, large pads are applied along the site of vein removal and covered with an inelastic bandage.
- An elastic bandage or compression stockings are then applied.

Postprocedural Care

- Refer to Exhibit 19.3 for basic postprocedural care.
- If patient is having bleeding, then gentle pressure is applied. Leg elevation for 5 to 10 minutes post procedure can be useful.
- Pain control.

Complications

- Pain
- Varicose vein recurrence
- Edema
- Bruising bleeding
- Hyperpigmentation
- Tissue necrosis
- Thrombophlebitis
- DVT
- Telangiectasia
- Sensory deficits

Follow-Up/Patient Education

- Follow up with interventional radiology in 4 to 6 weeks post procedure.
- Patient should ambulate for 15 to 20 minutes several times a day.

- Dressings can be removed in 1 to 2 days.
- Compression stockings should be worn for 1 to 3 weeks post procedure. Patient may develop numbness in the lower extremities due to compression stockings; this can require removal of stockings and using lower pressure stockings.
- Avoid heavy lifting and strenuous activities for 1 to 2 weeks. Patient can usually return to normal activities in 3 to 7 days.
- Ultrasound to evaluate for DVT is performed initially to exclude the presence of a DVT, a rare complication. Ultrasound follow-up in 1 to 4 weeks after treatment is recommended by the Union of Internationale de Phlebologie (UIP) to determine the success of therapy and evaluate for recurrence of varicose veins.
- Bruising and hyperpigmentation usually resolve in several months.
- Follow up with interventional radiology in 4 to 6 weeks post procedure.
- Discharge instructions should advise patient to seek medical attention if having swelling at puncture site or swelling of the extremity suggesting DVT.

Venography/Vein Mapping

Introduction

- Venography is a procedure used for assessing the anatomy and flow in veins.
- Access is obtained distal or upstream to the region of interest and contrast agent injected under fluoroscopy to visualize the region of interest.

Indications

- Evaluation for DVT
- Venous malformation
- Evaluation for tumor encasement of venous structures
- Evaluation for fistula creation

Contraindications

- Pregnancy

Preprocedure Care

- Refer to Exhibit 19.1 for preprocedural care.

Anesthesia

- Procedure is usually performed with local anesthesia and minimal sedation.
- Moderate sedation can also be used.

Intraprocedural Care

- Refer to Exhibit 19.2 for intraprocedural care.
- Patient is placed on fluoroscopy table, usually in supine position.
- Ultrasound may be used for identifying the venous site initially and then fluoroscopy.
- For DVT, dorsum veins of the foot are used for access and injection.
- Tourniquet or blood pressure cuff can be utilized to prevent filling of superficial veins.

Postprocedural Care

- Refer to Exhibit 19.3 for postprocedural care.

Complications

- Entry site hematoma
- Contrast extravasation into subcutaneous soft tissue
- Contrast-induced nephropathy
- Contrast reaction
- Infection
- Thrombophlebitis
- Refer to Chapter 12, Iodinated Contrast Adverse Events, for the treatment of contrast reactions.

Follow-Up/Patient Education

- Outpatient follow-up in 4 to 6 weeks

Fast Facts

- The goal of ablation and sclerotherapy is to cause fibrosis of the varicose vein: NSAIDs can interfere with this process and, therefore, should be avoided.
- Patients are at risk of developing DVT after the procedure. An ultrasound to evaluate for DVT is usually performed within the first week after the procedure.

Sclerotherapy

Introduction

- Sclerotherapy is an alternative treatment for varicose veins.
- A sclerosing agent is then injected into the abnormal veins while avoiding damage to other vessels. This agent causes endothelial and vessel wall damage, resulting in obliteration of the vein into a thread of connective tissue.

- Ultrasound can be employed in this procedure to visualize and access the abnormal veins.

Indications

- Symptomatic small varicose veins
- Spider veins
- Remnant veins after ablative therapy and phlebectomy
- For cosmetic purposes

Contraindications

- Allergy to sclerosing agents
- Vein thrombosis or acute thrombophlebitis
- Hypercoagulable state
- Peripheral vascular disease
- Patent foramen ovale or other cardiac shunts to avoid paradoxical emboli
- Immobility
- Pregnancy

Preprocedural Care

- Refer to Exhibit 19.1 for basic preprocedural care.

Anesthesia

- Procedure is usually performed with perivenous tumescent anesthesia.

Intraprocedural Care

- Refer to Exhibit 19.2 for basic intraprocedural care.
- The positioning of the patient depends on site of sclerotherapy.
- Ultrasound can be used to access the veins.

Postprocedural Care

- Refer to Exhibit 19.3 for basic postprocedural care.
- Pain control with acetaminophen or codeine. NSAIDs should be avoided because these medications inhibit the inflammatory process that is part of the goal of therapy to treat the varicose veins.

Complications

- Anaphylaxis
- Pain
- Bruising
- Hyperpigmentation
- Tissue necrosis

PART IV   INTERVENTIONAL RADIOLOGY

- Thrombophlebitis
- DVT
- Stroke
- Visual changes
- Cough

Follow-Up/Patient Education

- Patient should ambulate for 15 to 20 minutes several times a day.
- Compression stockings should be worn for 1 to 3 weeks post procedure.
- Avoid heavy lifting and strenuous activities for 1 to 2 weeks. Patient can usually return to normal activities in 3 to 7 days.
- Ultrasound to evaluate for DVT is performed in 1 week to evaluate for DVT.
- Follow up with interventional radiology in 4 to 6 weeks post procedure.

Reference

Wang, M., & Sharma, A. K. (2019). Varicose veins. *Journal of Radiology Nursing, 38*(3), 150–154. doi:10.1016/j.jradnu.2019.04.004

20

Central Venous Catheters, Implantable Devices, and Dialysis Access

Nana Ohene Baah and Ashwani Kumar Sharma

Central venous catheters and implantable devices are placed to allow access to large veins for therapeutic treatment and diagnostic evaluation. Image guidance available in interventional radiology (IR) allows for safer placement of these catheters.

Chronic renal disease is characterized by a loss of renal function over a period of time. There are five stages of renal disease, with eventual failure requiring dialysis and/or transplant. Care of patients is complex, with IR playing an important role in the delivery of that care.

In this chapter, you will discover:

1. Central venous catheters and implantable devices
2. EKG monitoring during procedure
3. Maintenance of the central venous catheters and implantable devices
4. Stages of chronic kidney disease
5. Pulse assessments pre and post procedure
6. Procedural complications

CENTRAL VENOUS CATHETERS AND IMPLANTABLE DEVICES

Introduction

- Central venous catheters and implantable devices are placed to allow access to large veins for therapeutic treatment and diagnostic evaluation.
- Catheters used in this procedure vary in size, number of lumens, sites of insertion, and duration of use. They include tunneled small-bore central venous catheters, tunneled and nontunneled large-bore dialysis catheters, nontunneled venous catheters, and peripherally inserted venous catheters.
- Implantable devices (mediport) vary in size and number of lumens/septa. Because they are implanted, they are indicated for longer-term use and are traditionally placed for chemotherapy, plasmapheresis, and sometimes total parenteral nutrition.
- Image guidance by IR allows for a faster and safer insertion of such catheters and implantable devices.
- Access is obtained into the large central veins such as the internal jugular vein, subclavian vein, and femoral vein using ultrasound; then, fluoroscopy is used to guide wire positioning and ultimate catheter placement at the cavoatrial junction. Peripheral vein options include the basilic and the paired brachial veins. The cephalic vein is rarely used.

Indications

- Administration of intravenous (IV) fluids, especially for rapid infusion or in patients requiring massive volume repletion
- Administration of medications, especially drugs that cannot be administered peripherally such as vasopressors, chemotherapeutic drugs, and antibiotics
- Blood products
- Total parental nutrition
- Plasmapheresis
- Hemodialysis
- Hemodynamic monitoring
- Poor peripheral venous access
- Repeated or frequent blood sampling

Contraindications

- Cellulitis at the site of insertion
- Bacteremia/septicemia

- Thrombosis of the veins chosen for insertion
- Hyperkalemia greater than 6 mmol/L may require a femoral venous approach due to cardiac wall instability.
- Severe coagulopathy warrants a nontunneled placement.

Preprocedural Care

- Refer to Exhibit 19.1 for basic preprocedural care.

Anesthesia

- Procedure usually performed with moderate sedation and local anesthesia.

Intraprocedural Care

- Refer to Exhibit 19.2 for basic intraprocedural care.
- Place patient on fluoroscopy table, usually in supine position.
- Administer prophylactic antibiotics if patient is not receiving intravenous antibiotics, usually first-generation cephalosporin such as cefazolin IV; alternatives include vancomycin for patients with a penicillin allergy.
- Preliminary sonographic evaluation for patency is performed. The right internal jugular vein is usually preferred for ultrasound-guided access, followed by the left side. Rarely, the subclavian veins and the femoral veins are utilized. Femoral vein sites are typically not preferred due to a higher association with central line-associated bloodstream infections (CLABSI). Fluoroscopy may then be used to direct the catheter, over a guiding wire, into the distal superior vena cava or the right atrium.
- For the implantable device, a subcutaneous pocket is made about 1 to 2 cm below the clavicle for implantation. Subsequently, a connecting catheter is tunneled to the access site, and the catheter tip is then guided into the superior vena cava/right atrium through a sheath. The incisions site is closed with sutures.
- Apply protective skin disk such as chlorhexidine disk and clear sterile occlusive dressing to the catheter site. There are usually two skin incisions made for tunneled catheter central lines: The central venous site should be dressed with gauze and clear occlusive dressing.
- Flush catheter ports with normal saline to clear them from blood.
- Catheters and implantable devices are usually locked with heparin. If patient is allergic to heparin, use tPA.

Pay special attention to EKG monitoring when catheters are placed within the cardiac chambers due to possibility of arrhythmia.

Postprocedural Care

- Refer to Exhibit 19.3 for basic postprocedural care.
- Assess for shortness of breath, as this can be a sign of pneumothorax.
- Use postprocedural chest x-ray to evaluate for pneumothorax, other complications related to the procedure, and positioning of the catheter if fluoroscopy is not utilized during initial placement.

Complications

- Bleeding, infection, or injury to the surrounding structures at the insertion site such as nerves or arterial placement.

Follow-Up/Patient Education for Central Venous Catheters

- Catheters require routine dressing changes and instillation with heparin or TPA after use to prevent thrombosis.
- Routinely flush catheters and implantable devices after access/completion therapy.
- Remove catheters when they are no longer needed. This can be done at bedside or as an outpatient with or without minimal sedation. Implantable devices require some subcuticular dissection for retrieval; thus, they are typically performed in a sterile environment/angiography suite under moderate sedation

Follow-Up/Patient Education for Implantable Devices

- Routine outpatient follow-up in 1 week to assess port site. The port can be accessed during this period, if needed.
- Remove implantable devices when they are no longer needed. Removal requires an outpatient procedure with moderate sedation to remove all the port components.

PROCEDURAL CARE FOR PATIENTS WITH CHRONIC KIDNEY DISEASE

Chronic renal disease is a worldwide health problem with rising incidence and prevalence resulting in poor outcomes and high cost. In 2000, the National Kidney Foundation (NKF) Kidney Disease Outcome Quality Initiative (KDOQI) Advisory Board approved the development of clinical practice guidelines to define chronic kidney disease and classify stages in the progression of chronic kidney disease (see Table 20.1). The Work Group charged with developing the guidelines consisted of experts in nephrology, pediatric nephrology, epidemiology, laboratory medicine, nutrition, social work, gerontology, and family medicine. Definition of chronic renal disease as defined by KDOQI workgroup:

- Kidney damage for ≥3 months, as defined by structural or functional abnormalities of the kidney, with or without decreased estimated glomerular filtration rate (eGFR), manifest by either
  - Pathological abnormalities
  - Markers of kidney damage, including abnormalities in the composition of the blood or urine, or abnormalities in imaging tests
- GFR <60 mL/min/1.73 m² for ≥3 months, with or without kidney damage

Table 20.1

Chronic Kidney Disease Classification		
Stage	**eGFR**	**Intervention**
Stage 1	≥90 mL/min/1.73 m²	Diagnosis and treatment of the primary disease
Stage 2	60–89 mL/min/1.73 m²	Monitoring the disease
Stage 3	30–59 mL/min/1.73 m²	Primary disease complication management
Stage 4	15–29 mL/min/1.73 m²	Getting ready for kidney replacement therapy
Stage 5	15 mL/min/1.73 m²	Dialysis and/or kidney transplant

- Check and document pulses of the major arteries in the arm before and after the procedure.
- Heparin is given during the procedure to prevent fistula thrombosis.
- Patient may require dialysis after the procedure depending on labs and fluid status.

The National Kidney Foundation Kidney Disease Outcomes Quality Initiative guidelines indicate tunneled cuffed venous catheters (TCVCs) for temporary venous access that is expected to be required for longer than 3 weeks and may serve as bridging devices during maturation of newly placed arteriovenous fistulas or as the final option in patients in whom fistulas and grafts have failed.

Long-term dialysis access is created via the surgical construction of an arteriovenous fistula or shunt graft. The KDOQI document recommends that the order of preference for the site of shunt/fistula should be radiocephalic wrist fistula followed by brachiocephalic elbow fistula and transposed brachial-basilic vein fistula. An arteriovenous graft should only be considered if arteriovenous fistula (AVF) creation is not possible.

Regular assessment of AVFs should be performed to detect hemodynamically significant stenosis and decrease the incidence of thrombosis of fistula and improve long-term patency. Direct flow measurements and duplex ultrasound are the preferred methods of surveillance. If there is a decrease in flow rates, intervention with fistulogram is warranted.

DIALYSIS FISTULAS AND DIALYSIS ATRIOVENOUS GRAFT

Indications

- Diagnostic fistulogram assesses maturation of atriovenous fistula: Usually performed 6 weeks after the creation of the fistula.
- Therapeutic fistulogram is the assessment of malfunctioning fistula due to anastomotic stenosis, venous outflow stenosis, or fistula thrombosis.

Contraindications

- Infection
- Right to left heart shunt

Preprocedural Care

- Refer to Exhibit 19.1 for basic preprocedural care.

Anesthesia

- Moderate sedation and local anesthesia

Intraprocedural Care

- Refer to Exhibit 19.2 for basic intraprocedural care.
- Patient placed on fluoroscopy table, usually in supine position.
- Heparin 3,000 units intravenous (IV) is given initially and as needed during the procedure.
- Nitroglycerin should be available in case of vasospasm.
- Ultrasound used for identifying the access site initially and then fluoroscopy is used.

Fast Facts

Pulses in the major arteries of the arm should be checked and documented before and after the fistulogram procedure.

Postprocedural Care

- Refer to Exhibit 19.3 for basic postprocedural care.
- Patient may require dialysis after the procedure depending on labs.

Complications

- Volume overload can result from the fluids administered during the procedure, especially in these patients with impaired renal function.
  - Evaluate for shortness of breath and auscultate for lung crackles.
  - Patient may need dialysis for fluid overload.

- Shortness of breath could be caused by a pulmonary embolism.
- Arterial embolism in the forearm may occur.
  - Assessment for pulses and limb ischemia is therefore important post procedure.
- Contrast reaction, infection, hematoma, or bleeding may occur.

Follow-Up/Patient Education

- Outpatient follow-up in 4 to 6 weeks.

Fast Facts

Patient may require dialysis after the procedure depending on labs and fluid status.

21

Portal Hypertension and Transvenous Interventions

Nana Ohene Baah

Liver disease and liver failure can be caused by chronic alcohol consumption, viral hepatitis, and chronic fat deposits, among other causes. Life-threatening effects can occur with liver disease, which require specialized treatment to preserve a quality of life for the patient.

Gonadal venous congestion can occur in both men and women. This can cause infertility and/or pain. Interventional radiology (IR) procedures are minimally invasive and can help alleviate these symptoms.

In this chapter, you will discover:

1. Introduction to cirrhosis and sequelae of portal hypertension
2. Management of sequelae of portal hypertension
3. Paracentesis and thoracentesis
4. Pelvic congestion syndrome
5. Embolization of variceles
6. Embolization of gonadal vein

CIRRHOSIS AND PORTAL HYPERTENSION

Introduction

- Cirrhosis is a terminal liver ailment resulting from chronic hepatocellular injury. It leads to irreversible scarring and liver failure.
- Chronic alcohol use, viral hepatitis, and chronic fat deposition in the liver are common causes of liver failure.
- Severe distortion of the hepatic parenchymal and portal vascular architecture in cirrhosis creates abnormally high portal pressures and portal hypertension.
- Potentially life-threatening complications include:
  a. Variceal bleeding
  b. Ascites
  c. Hepatorenal syndrome
  d. Hepatic hydrothorax
  e. Encephalopathy
  f. Enterocolopathic hemorrhage
- Paracentesis, thoracentesis, and transjugular intrahepatic portosystemic shunts (TIPSS) are some interventions to manage complications of portal hypertension.

TRANSJUGULAR INTRAHEPATIC PORTOSYSTEMIC SHUNTS (TIPSS)

Introduction

- TIPSS is a percutaneous procedure that creates a vascular shunt between the portal venous system and the systemic venous circulation to alleviate portal hypertension.
- In most circumstances, access is obtained in the right internal jugular vein.
- Catheter is advanced into the hepatic veins. Venogram can be performed.
- A shunt is created between a hepatic vein and a portal vein branch.

Indications

- Prevention of esophageal variceal bleeding
- Recurrent cirrhotic ascites
- Pleural effusion due to hepatic disease

Contraindications

- Severe right heart failure
- Severe or progressive liver failure

- Hepatic encephalopathy that has failed medical management
- Allergy to stent components
- Sepsis/bacteremia

Preprocedural Care

- Refer to Exhibit 19.1 for basic preprocedural care.

Anesthesia

- The procedure is usually performed under general anesthesia.
- Moderate or deep sedation can also be used.

Intraprocedural Care

- Refer to Exhibit 19.2 for basic intraprocedural care.
- Prophylactic antibiotics, usually ceftriaxone or Zosyn. Alternatives include ciprofloxacin or vancomycin.
- Venous access for TIPSS is usually via the right internal jugular vein.
- Ultrasound for vein access, then fluoroscopy during the procedure.
- A pressure transducer is needed.
  - Calibrate to zero prior to the procedure.
  - Pressure measurements before and after TIPSS creation should include right atrial, central venous pressure, hepatic vein, and hepatic wedge pressures.
  - Right atrial pressure should be less than 10 mmHg.
  - Portal systemic pressure gradient should be less than 12 mmHg in variceal bleeding.

Fast Facts

Portal venous pressure is the blood pressure in the hepatic portal vein and is normally between 5 and 10 mmHg.

Postprocedural Care

- Refer to Exhibit 19.3 for postprocedural care.
- Assess for shortness of breath, as patient may develop pulmonary edema and require diuresis.
- Assess for mental status, as patients are at risk of developing hepatic encephalopathy.
- Patient requires at least 24-hour observation post procedure.

Complications

- Entry-site hematoma
- Fever
- Contrast-induced nephropathy
- Hemoperitoneum
- Haemobilia
- Gallbladder injury
- Liver infarction
- Hepatic encephalopathy
- Stent thrombosis or stenosis
- Recurrent variceal bleeding

Follow-Up/Patient Education

- Outpatient follow-up in 4 to 6 weeks and an ultrasound exam at 3 months to evaluate the patency of the shunt (TIPSS may become stenosed or occluded.)

PARACENTESIS

Introduction

- Paracentesis involves the removal of fluid accumulated in the peritoneal cavity for diagnostic or therapeutic purposes.
- Peritoneal fluid is analyzed to diagnose infection or metastasis to the peritoneal cavity.
  - Tests may include cell count, cell differential, albumin, lactate dehydrogenase (LDH), and cultures.
- A therapeutic paracentesis relieves tense ascites, which are commonly found in cirrhotic patients.
  - A larger gauge needle is used to remove as much fluid as tolerated by the patient.
  - Several different needles can be used; typically, an 18 gauge is preferred.
  - Newer devices include a one-step needle, which has a removable needle inside a catheter, and a valved one-step needle.
- The procedure can be performed at bedside or in the radiology department (for more complicated patients).

Indications

- Evaluation of new-onset ascites

- Diagnostic testing in patients with signs of an infection of the peritoneal cavity such as fever, abdominal pain, abdominal tenderness, or leukocytosis
- Testing of peritoneal fluid in patients with preexisting ascites

Contraindications

- If benefits outweigh risks, paracentesis is always performed.
- Relative contraindications include disseminated intravascular coagulation and massive ileus with bowel distention.
- Elevated international normalized ratio (INR) or coagulopathy is *not* a contraindication for paracentesis.

Preprocedural Care

- Refer to Exhibit 19.1 for basic preprocedural care.

Anesthesia

- Typically performed with local anesthesia but can use moderate sedation

Intraprocedural Care

- Refer to Exhibit 19.2 for basic intraprocedural care.
- Ultrasound is performed to identify a safe acoustic window to optimize drainage.
- Radiologist marks the entry site, which is usually in the left lower abdominal quadrant.
- Peritoneal fluid collected for analysis should be labeled per organizational policy.

Special Considerations

- Start colloid replacement with a 5% or 25% solution after 3 to 5 L of fluid is removed.
- Patients not receiving albumin are more likely to show signs of hemodynamic deterioration and worsening renal function.

Fast Facts

If more than 3 to 5 L of fluid is removed, 6 to 8 g of albumin for every liter of fluid removed is given to prevent hypotension.

Postprocedural Care

■ Refer to Exhibit 19.3 for basic postprocedural care.

Complications

■ Leakage of peritoneal fluid, infection, bleeding, and injury to bowel can occur.
■ For a peritoneal fluid leak, an occlusive dressing or topical adhesive can be applied.
  ■ If the leak continues, an ostomy bag can be placed to quantify the fluid, and further treatment options can be discussed with a physician.
  ■ Intraperitoneal infections are rare from the procedure: A persistent leak can lead cellulitis at the puncture site.
■ Bleeding from an injured artery or vein can be severe.
  ■ Abdomen pain, tenderness, and hypotension should raise concern.

Follow-Up/Patient Education

■ Patient follows up with primary care physician after procedure.
■ Patient should contact primary care physician if puncture site demonstrates signs of infection or if the fluid reaccumulates.

THORACENTESIS

Introduction

■ Fluid or air in the pleural space may be the result of trauma, hepatic hydrothorax from cirrhosis, heart failure, or pulmonary diseases such as cancer or infection.
■ A thoracentesis allows removal of air (pneumothorax) and/or pleural fluid for diagnostic or therapeutic purposes.
■ When bilateral thoracentesis is desired, one side is performed, and patient is monitored for complications prior to performing the procedure on the contralateral side.
■ A pleural drain catheter can be placed for therapeutic drainage after the procedure.

Indications

■ *Diagnostic thoracentesis* determines whether fluid in the pleural space is the result of lung malignancy, parapneumonic effusion due to infection, or a simple effusion due to altered hemodynamics as seen in cirrhosis or heart failure.

■ *Therapeutic thoracentesis* drains significant pleural effusions causing dyspnea or hypoxia.
■ Also performed for draining parapneumonic effusion, hemothorax, or pneumothorax.

Contraindications

■ Uncorrectable coagulopathy

Preprocedural Care

■ Refer to Exhibit 19.1 for basic preprocedural care.

Anesthesia

■ Procedure usually performed with minimal sedation and local anesthesia.
■ Moderate sedation is rarely used.

Intraprocedural Care

■ Refer to Exhibit 19.2 for basic intraprocedural care.
■ Patient placed in the upright sitting position while leaning on the table.
  ■ Alternatively, the patient can be placed in the lateral decubitus position.
  ■ In certain cases, with pneumothorax or loculated effusion, the procedure may be performed with CT guidance or fluoroscopy guidance, and the patient positioning should be confirmed with the operator.
■ Ultrasound is usually used for identifying the access site.
  ■ A limited ultrasound exam is performed for identification of optimal fluid pocket and the radiologist marks the entry site, usually at the sixth or seventh intercostal rib space at the midaxillary line or back.
■ Special attention should be paid to respiratory rate and oxygen saturation due to risk of pneumothorax.
■ Fluid sample may be aspirated and sent for diagnostic evaluation.
■ A tunneled pleural catheter can be left in place if long-term drainage is desired.
  ■ *Parapneumonic* and exudative effusions usually require a larger bore drain that is at least 12 to 14 French catheters.

- ■ Transudative effusions can be drained with an 8 to 10 French catheters.
- ■ Pleural drains need to be connected to chest tube system to allow for drainage.
- ■ Entry site into the thorax is covered with occlusive dressing such as gauze coated with white petroleum jelly.

Postprocedural Care

- ■ Refer to Exhibit 19.3 for postprocedural care.
- ■ Pay special attention to respiratory rate and oxygen saturation.
  - ■ Check for dyspnea and lung sounds on physical exam as patient may develop pneumothorax.
- ■ Upright chest radiograph is performed to evaluate for pneumothorax.

Complications

- ■ Pneumothorax
- ■ Infection
- ■ Bleeding
- ■ Drainage catheter malfunction

Fast Facts

Drainage of fluid should be limited to a maximum of 1 to 1.5 L of fluid in one day to prevent reexpansion pulmonary edema. The amount of fluid drained during the procedure should be communicated to the receiving nurse.

Follow-Up/Patient Education

- ■ Outpatient follow-up in 2 to 4 weeks.
- ■ Patients with pleural catheter require instructions on outpatient drainage.
  - ■ A pleural catheter has a bulb that is compressed and connected to the chest tube for drainage when patient feels fluid accumulating in their pleural cavity. The bulb fills with fluid as it drains the fluid.
- ■ Patients with pleural drains are followed clinically by recording output and with radiographs to determine when the pleural drain can be removed.

PELVIC CONGESTION SYNDROME, VARICOCELE, AND GONADAL VEIN EMBOLIZATION

Introduction

- Tortuous dilatation of the gonadal veins can result in incompetent valves, compromised venous drainage of the gonads, and chronic abdominopelvic pain.

- In females, this condition is referred to as *pelvic congestion syndrome*. It typically involves the ovarian veins and presents with dull-aching deep pelvic pain that frequently affects the left side. This entity may also be associated with dyspareunia and thigh and vulvar varices.

- The male equivalent of pelvic congestion syndrome is *varicoceles*, characterized by tortuous dilatation of the pampiniform venous plexus in the scrotum due to incompetent valves in the internal spermatic vein.
  - Similar symptoms are described in males, including dull-aching scrotal pain more commonly affecting the left side.
  - Varicoceles can result in dysfunctional sperm and presents a potentially treatable cause of male infertility.
  - Gonadal vein embolization treats pelvic congestion syndrome in females and varicoceles in males. In females, the ovarian vein is embolized, and, in males, embolization of the internal spermatic vein is performed for treatment.

- Gonadal vein embolization is performed by gaining access to the right femoral vein or right internal jugular vein, a wire is then placed, and a catheter is advanced to the internal spermatic vein or the ovarian vein. The target vessel is then occluded using embolization coils in conjunction with a sclerosant such as sodium tetradecyl sulfate or liquid glue embolic agent.

Indications

- In males:
  - Scrotal pain
  - Infertility
  - Recurrent varicocele
  - Testicular atrophy in pediatric patients
- In females:
  - Chronic, dull, deep pelvic pain and pressure that may be positional or worsen with movement
  - Thigh and vulvar varices
  - Vulvar point tenderness

Contraindications

- Severe coagulopathy
- Severe contrast reaction

Preprocedural Care

- Refer to Exhibit 19.1 for basic preprocedural care.

Anesthesia

- Gonadal embolization is performed under conscious sedation.

Intraprocedural Care

- Refer to Exhibit 19.2 for basic intraprocedural care.
- Place patient in supine position.
- Ultrasound may be used for identifying the vein initially, and then fluoroscopy is performed.

Postprocedural Care

- Refer to Exhibit 19.3 for basic postprocedural care.

Complications

- A small percentage of patients will develop:
  - Back pain, which can be treated with acetaminophen.
  - Scrotal or vulvar edema, which can be managed with nonsteroidal anti-inflammatory drugs (NSAIDs) and a heating pad.
- Migration of embolization coils into the central venous system and venous perforation, which is usually self-limiting.

Follow Up/Patient Education

- Patient follows up with primary care physician after procedure and with interventional radiology in 4 to 6 weeks.
- Provide discharge instructions with contact information.

Fast Facts

Prior abdominopelvic imaging with contrast (CT or MRI) is necessary to exclude other causes of gonadal vein dilatation such as compression from abdominal masses or abnormal vascular course.

22

Vertebral Body Augmentation and Percutaneous Ablation

Nana Ohene Baah and
Ashwani Kumar Sharma

Minimally invasive procedures assist patients in reaching a higher quality of life. Vertebral augmentation uses a special bone cement to stabilize fractures and ultimately decrease pain. Fallopian tube recanalization is a minimally invasive procedure that opens an occluded fallopian tube in women who experience subfertility.

Minimally invasive percutaneous ablation techniques have gained popularity in the treatment of a variety of patient lesions and tumors. Different energy sources and techniques allow the proceduralist to provide the most effective treatment available for each particular diagnosis.

In this chapter, you will discover:

1. Care of the patient undergoing vertebral augmentation procedures
2. Infertility treatment for fallopian tube occlusion
3. The fundamentals of ablation
4. Differences between thermal and cryoablation
5. Applications of ablation

VERTEBROPLASTY AND KYPHOPLASTY

Introduction

- Compression fractures of the spinal vertebra can cause significant back pain.
- Vertebroplasty is a procedure for stabilizing the vertebra by advancing a needle and injecting cement into the vertebral body.
- Kyphoplasty is a more involved procedure with a cannula placed into the vertebral pedicle. The cannula is used for drilling of the vertebra to create a channel for ballooning and creating a cavity in the vertebral body. This cavity is then filled with cement.
- Both procedures are performed with fluoroscopy.
- Patient should have prior imaging such as spinal radiographs, CT of the spine, or MRI of the spine to determine the target vertebra for treatment.
- MRI of the lumbar spine determines the acuity of the fracture because acute/subacute fractures with MRI findings of marrow edema demonstrate better clinical outcomes after augmentation.

Indications

- Pain associated with vertebral body compression fracture (acute/subacute)

Contraindications

- Allergy to cement
- Systemic infection or bacteremia
- Fractures causing spinal canal compromise or spinal cord myelopathy
- Coagulopathy

Preprocedural Care

- Refer to Exhibit 19.1 for basic preprocedural care.

Anesthesia

- Procedure usually performed with moderate sedation and local anesthesia

Intraprocedural Care

- Refer to Exhibit 19.2 for basic intraprocedural care.
- Patient is placed on fluoroscopy table, usually in prone position.
- Prophylactic antibiotics are given with Ancef 1 g IV.
- Special care of room temperature and cement temperature must occur following manufacturer's recommendations during procedure.

Fast Facts

MRI of the lumbar spine is especially important in determining the acuity of the fracture. Acute/subacute fractures with MRI findings of marrow edema demonstrate better clinical outcomes after augmentation (Zhou, Meng, Zhu, Zhu, & Yuan, 2019).

Postprocedural Care

- Refer to Exhibit 19.3 for basic postprocedural care.

Follow-Up

- Complications include:
  - Bleeding
  - Infection
  - Pneumothorax when the procedure involves the thoracic vertebra
  - Nerve damage or motor neuropathy
  - Pulmonary emboli from the cement
  - Fractures of vertebra adjacent to treated vertebra

FALLOPIAN TUBE RECANALIZATION

Introduction

- Fallopian tube occlusion results in infertility. Fallopian tube recanalization is an image-guided intervention for relieving blockages of the fallopian tubes.
- Prior to recanalization, a hysterosalpingogram is performed by inserting a catheter through the cervix and injecting contrast dye in the uterine cavity. Upon confirmation of fallopian

tubal occlusion, a second catheter is used to cannulate the fallopian tube.
- Hysterosalpingogram is then repeated to check for patency of the fallopian tubes.

Indications

- Infertility due to fallopian tube occlusion
- Recanalization after tubal ligation reversal

Contraindications

- Pelvic infection
- Intrauterine adhesions
- Distal tubal occlusion
- Pregnancy

Preprocedural Care

- Refer to Exhibit 19.1 for basic preprocedural care.

Anesthesia

- Procedure usually performed with minimal sedation. Moderate sedation can be used.

Intraprocedural Care

- Refer to Exhibit 19.2 for basic intraprocedural care.
- Prophylaxis antibiotics are usually given.
- Patient placed on fluoroscopy table in lithotomy position.
- Vaginal speculum is inserted, and cervix is prepped in sterile fashion.

Postprocedural Care

- Refer to Exhibit 19.3 for basic postprocedural care.
- Assess for abdominal pain as severe abdominal pain may indicate a complication such as tubal perforations.

Complications

- Pelvic infection
- Tubal perforation
- Ectopic pregnancy

Follow-Up/Patient Education

- Outpatient follow-up in 4 to 6 weeks.
- Vaginal spotting and cramping for the first 2 days is expected.
- Do not engage in sex or put anything in the vagina for 48 hours post procedure, including tampons.

Fallopian tube tecanalization on YouTube: https://www.youtube.com/watch?v=rffclVvkNYE.

ABLATION: MICROWAVE ABLATION, CRYOABLATION, OR RADIOFREQUENCY ABLATION

Introduction

- Minimally invasive techniques of percutaneous ablation have gained acceptance in the treatment and/or palliation of small tumors.
- *Thermal energy* is utilized with microwave ablation and radiofrequency ablation for therapeutic benefit. However, extremely *cold temperatures* are employed by cryoablation techniques to destroy target tumor lesions.
- These minimally invasive techniques offer the benefit of preservation of organ function, shorter recovery time, and reduced mortality and morbidity.
- *Microwave ablation*, the newest ablative phenomenon, uses electromagnetic waves within the microwave frequency spectrum for therapeutic benefits. In essence, under ultrasound or CT guidance, a microwave probe attached to a microwave generator is advanced into a soft tissue or bone tumor lesion. The electromagnetic waves generate heat, which induce cellular death via coagulative necrosis.
- *Radiofrequency ablation* uses a needle electrode under an alternating current to generate a high amount of heat, which incites cellular death via coagulative necrosis. The needle electrode is advanced under imaging guidance until it reaches the proper position in the target tissue. Several passes are taken if the lesion is larger than the probe's ablation diameter in order to achieve the ablative end goal.
- In *cryoablation*, hollow needles are placed simultaneously under image guidance into the target tissue with larger tumors requiring more needles. Liquid argon or carbon dioxide is then used to

rapidly cool the uninsulated tip of the needle for a set amount of time. Several cycles of freezing, thawing, and refreezing occur to induce cellular death via disruption of cellular organelles and membranes.

- Typical candidates for these procedures are patients with several small lesions or patients with comorbidities precluding traditional surgical resection.
- Interventional radiologists usually treat tumors located in the liver or kidney with these procedures, but breast, prostate, bone, and lung lesions can also be treated. Radiofrequency ablation is especially useful in treating spinal metastasis for pain palliation. Benign bone tumors such as osteoid osteomas and osteoblastomas are also commonly treated for symptomatic relief.

Indications

- Palliative care for hepatocellular carcinoma
- Treatment of liver metastasis
- Small renal lesions with high suspicion for malignancy
- Vertebral body and other bony metastasis
- Osteoid osteomas and osteoblastomas

Contraindications

- Tumor lesion located close to a main biliary duct
- Intrahepatic biliary duct dilation
- Untreatable coagulopathy

Preprocedural Care

- Refer to Exhibit 19.1 for basic preprocedural care.

Anesthesia

- Radiofrequency ablation and microwave ablation are performed under general anesthesia. Cryoablation may be performed under moderate sedation.

Intraprocedural Care

- Refer to Exhibit 19.2 for basic intraprocedural care.
- Check with physician for patient positioning. Ablation typically performed with patient in prone position.
- Ultrasound or CT guidance is used to determine the best approach to the tumor.

Postprocedural Care

- Refer to Exhibit 19.3 for basic postprocedural care.
- Bed rest is advised for 2 hours, and the patient is monitored as inpatient for 24 hours.
- Monitor urine output.
    - If patient has discomfort, inability to urinate, or no urine output for 8 hours post surgery, consider a bedside bladder scan.
- Physician may order the placement of a urinary catheter.

Complications

- Minor side effects from the procedure include pain at the ablation site and fever.
- Major complications may include:
    - Intraperitoneal hemorrhage (abdominal pain, tenderness, hypotension)
    - Intestinal perforation (rigid abdomen with tenderness)
    - Pneumothorax (shortness of breath)
    - Hemorrhage
    - Urinoma
    - Hematuria from intraparenchymal pseudoaneurysm or arteriovenous fistula

Follow-Up/Patient Education

- Follow up with interventional radiologist in 4 to 6 weeks.
- Follow-up imaging in 10 to 12 weeks is recommended to evaluate interval changes for treated lesions.
- Patient should contact primary care physician if puncture site demonstrates signs of infection or if having swelling at puncture site, fevers, or chills.

Fast Facts

A rare complication of cryoablation is cryoshock, which can result in disseminated intravascular coagulopathy and multisystem organ failure.

Reference

Zhou, X., Meng, X., Zhu, H., Zhu, Y., & Yuan, W. (2019). Early versus late percutaneous kyphoplasty for treating osteoporotic vertebral compression fracture: A retrospective study. *Clinical Neurology and Neurosurgery, 180*, 101–105. doi:10.1016/j.clineuro.2019.03.029

23

Transarterial Access for Oncologic Interventions

Nana Ohene Baah and
Ashwani Kumar Sharma

Embolization is a procedure that places a synthetic material and/or chemotherapy directly into the blood vessel that feeds a tumor (benign or malignant). Blood flow is then cutoff, and when chemotherapy is utilized, the maximum effect of the medication can occur directly in the region of the cancerous tumor.

In this chapter, you will discover:

1. Radioembolization or chemoembolization hepatic malignancies
2. Uterine fibroid embolization
3. General patient care essentials

RADIOEMBOLIZATION OF HEPATIC MALIGNANCIES

Introduction

- This is an endovascular procedure for the treatment of primary hepatic malignancies or metastatic liver lesions.
- It is performed through percutaneous access through a femoral artery or a radial artery, and catheters are advanced to the hepatic arteries. Contrast is injected to select the vessel of interest.

- Tiny glass/resin beads instilled with the radioactive isotope Yttrium-90 are injected into the hepatic artery and are carried by blood flow to the distal arterioles supplying the tumor. They become trapped within these distal arterioles within the tumor where they emit beta particles to irradiate the tumor.
- Therapsheres and SIR-Spheres are two types of particles that are used for treatment.
- The goal of treatment is to shrink the tumor and preserve normal liver parenchyma and function.
- Preferred access is commonly via the right femoral artery, left femoral artery, or left radial artery.
- Patient usually has prior imaging of the liver lesion(s) using modalities such as CT or MRI prior to the procedure.

Indications

- Unresectable hepatocellular carcinoma
- Metastatic neoplasm to the liver

Contraindications

- Hepatopulmonary lung shunting of more than 20%
- Uncorrectable coagulopathy
- Poor candidate for chemoembolization
- Pregnancy
- Relative contraindications: poor hepatic function or biliary obstruction

Preprocedural Care

- Refer to Exhibit 19.1 for basic preprocedural care.

Anesthesia

- Procedure is usually performed with moderate sedation and local anesthesia.

Intraprocedural Care

- Refer to Exhibit 19.2 for basic intraprocedural care.
- Ultrasound may be used for identifying the venous site initially, and then fluoroscopy is utilized.
- Radioactive precautions should be in place.

Postprocedural Care

- Refer to Exhibit 19.3 for basic postprocedural care.
- Bed rest is advised for 2 hours.

- Monitor patients for *postembolization syndrome* characterized by abdominal pain, nausea, leukocytosis, and fever within the first 72 hours post procedure. This self-limiting phenomenon occurs as a result of an inflammatory response to acutely necrotizing tissue and is managed conservatively.

Fast Facts

Carefully monitor patients post procedure for *postembolization syndrome,* which is characterized by chills, rigors, leukocytosis, and hypotension. This is managed with supportive care using diphenhydramine, antipyretic, antiemetic, meperidine, and fluid resuscitation.

Complications

- Fatigue
- Abdominal pain
- Nausea
- Fever
- Contrast reaction
- Contrast-induced nephropathy
- Infection
- Pain at the access site
- Hematoma and bleeding at the arterial puncture site

Follow-Up/Patient Education

- Outpatient follow-up in 4 to 6 weeks.
- Provide discharge instructions with contact information. Advise patients that fever, chills, and malaise within the first 72 hours are self-limiting and should subside. If persistent, they should seek medical attention. Swelling and bleeding at the puncture site should also warrant emergent medical attention.

CHEMOEMBOLIZATION

Introduction

- Transcatheter arterial chemoembolization (TACE) treats tumors by selectively delivering chemotherapy to the lesion followed by occlusion of its blood supply.

- TACE is performed by gaining access to the artery supplying the tumor via a femoral arterial approach (right or left) or a left radial arterial approach.
  - A catheter is positioned with the tip in the feeding artery of the tumor, usually a branch of the hepatic artery.
  - A mixture of chemotherapeutic cocktail and an embolic agent, which may include small glass/resin beads or an embolic liquid called lipiodol, is injected via the feeding artery into the tumor. The embolic agent helps to enhance localization of the chemotherapy and decrease tumor blood flow to induce ischemic necrosis of the lesion.

Fast Facts

Commonly used chemotherapeutic drugs with chemoembolization are cisplatin, doxorubicin, and mitomycin C.

Indications

- Used as palliation of unresectable hepatocellular carcinomas.
- Treatment of lesions can maintain or downstage patients to within liver transplantation criteria.
- Treatment of metastatic lesions that are primarily confined to the liver.

Contraindications

- Poorly compensated advanced liver disease
- Poor performance status
- Large tumor burden
- Untreatable coagulopathy
- Severe contrast reaction

Preprocedural Care

- Refer to Exhibit 19.1 for basic preprocedural care.
- Hypotensive patients should be fluid resuscitated prior to procedure.
- Prophylactic antibiotics are given.

Anesthesia

- Chemoembolization is performed under moderate sedation.

Intraprocedural Care

- Refer to Exhibit 19.2 for basic intraprocedural care.
- Place patient in supine position.
- Access site is usually the right common femoral artery, left radial artery, or left common femoral artery.
- Prepare chemotherapeutic drugs for the physician.
- Prepare embolic agent; typically, embolization spheres.

Postprocedure Care

- Refer to Exhibit 19.3 for basic postprocedural care.
- Patients are placed on a PCA pump to control postoperative pain.
- Patient may be conservatively managed for postembolization syndrome with IV fluids, antipyretics, and antiemetics.

Complications

- Liver failure may occur in patients with poor preprocedure liver function.
  - Monitor for signs of encephalopathy, coagulopathy, and renal failure.
  - These may be managed with fluids, pressure support, and lactulose.
- Nontarget embolization of the gut, which can lead to bowel ischemia.

Follow-Up/Patient Education

- Patients follow up with interventional radiologist in 3 to 4 weeks.

UTERINE FIBROID EMBOLIZATION

Introduction

- This procedure is performed to obstruct blood flow in the uterine arteries for treatment of uterine fibroids. The procedure is performed to treat dysfunctional uterine bleeding and bulk symptoms due to large uterine fibroids. This procedure may also be performed emergently to control postpartum hemorrhage.
- It is performed through percutaneous access into a common femoral artery or left radial artery with catheter advanced to the uterine arteries. Contrast is injected to select the vessel of interest. Embolization materials, commonly glass/resin beads, are then deployed into the selected blood vessel to exclude blood supply

to the uterus and fibroids resulting in ischemic necrosis. As the fibroids shrink and calcify, the uterus fully recovers.

- Patients undergoing uterine artery embolization for symptomatic fibroids usually undergo imaging such as ultrasound or MRI in the preprocedural evaluation.

Indications

- Fibroids causing dysfunctional menstrual bleeding
- Fibroids causing pelvic pain or pelvic pressure
- Postpartum hemorrhage due to placental implantation anomalies

Contraindications

- Pregnancy is contraindication for fibroid embolization.

Preprocedural Care

- Refer to Exhibit 19.1 for basic preprocedural care.
- Foley catheter should be placed.

Anesthesia

- Procedure is usually performed with moderate sedation and local anesthesia. General anesthesia may be a consideration for some patients.

Intraprocedural Care

- Refer to Exhibit 19.2 for basic intraprocedural care.
- Patient is placed on fluoroscopy table usually in supine position.
- Patient usually receives prophylactic antibiotics such as cefazolin.
- Ultrasound may be used for identifying the access site initially, and then fluoroscopy is utilized.
- Heparin (1,000–5,000 units) is usually mixed with normal saline on the sterile tray.

Postprocedural Care

- Refer to Exhibit 19.3 for basic postprocedural care.
- Pain control is essential. Patient-controlled analgesia (PCA) pump may be used initially and then transitioned to nonsteroidal anti-inflammatory medications prior to discharge.
- Foley catheter should be removed 6 to 24 hours post procedure, and documentation of patient's ability to void should be performed prior to discharge.

- Nausea is a common side effect, and antiemetic medication should be ordered.

Complications

- Fibroid passage
- Contrast reaction
- Contrast-induced nephropathy
- Infection
- Pain at the access site
- Distal ischemia
- Arterial site complication such as hematoma
- Bleeding
- Pseudoaneurysm

Follow-Up/Patient Education

- Follow up with interventional radiology 1 week post procedure.
- Follow-up imaging with MRI or ultrasound can be performed 3 months post procedure to evaluate for treatment response.

Fast Facts

Uterine fibroid embolization is a minimally invasive procedure to help treat uterine fibroids in women who wish to conceive.

24

Transarterial Management of Trauma and Gastrointestinal Bleed

Nana Ohene Baah

Embolization procedures in interventional radiology (IR) obstruct blood flow for the treatment of an array of diseases and medical conditions, such as hemorrhage from traumatic injury, gastrointestinal bleeding, and vascular malformation. It can also treat tumors (see Chapter 23, Transarterial Access for Oncologic Interventions, on chemoembolization). This procedure is used for arterial bleeding, as venous bleeding is usually treated conservatively and does not require embolization.

In this chapter, you will discover:

1. Types of embolization procedures available for trauma and gastrointestinal bleeding
2. General and specific patient care essentials

TRAUMA AND SOLID ORGAN EMBOLIZATION

Introduction

- Performed to obstruct blood flow for treatment of an array of diseases and medical conditions, such as hemorrhage from traumatic injury, gastrointestinal bleeding, and vascular malformation.

- It can also treat tumors, which are discussed in other chapters.
- Venous bleeding is usually treated conservatively and does not require embolization.

Fast Facts

Arterial bleeding due to trauma can cause potentially life-threatening blood loss; these patients may require emergent IR intervention and volume resuscitation.

- Performed through percutaneous access into the blood vessels with the catheter advanced to the vessel of interest.
  - Contrast is injected to select the vessel of interest to perform a diagnostic angiogram. Vessel abnormalities are evaluated and, if warranted, embolization material is deployed into the selected blood vessel, followed by a contrast injection to check for success of the embolization.
- Different types of embolization materials are available, including coils, glue, alcohol, gelatin sponge, and microspheres.
- Imaging study, such as a CT scan, prior to the procedure can help identify the source of bleeding.
- Access is obtained into the femoral artery or left radial artery depending on the abnormality.

Indications

- Vascular injury due to trauma. Hemorrhage of gastrointestinal bleeding and arteriovenous malformations. Hemorrhage may need emergent embolization.
- Splenic artery embolization for splenic trauma and splenic artery pseudoaneurysm.
- Renal artery embolization for arterial injury due to renal trauma or iatrogenic from renal biopsy.
- Hepatic artery injury due to blunt trauma to the liver or iatrogenic from liver biopsy or biliary drainage catheter placement.
- Arterial injury due to skeletal fracture or muscular trauma.

Contraindications

- Hemodynamic instability; unstable trauma patients can be managed surgically or should be stabilized prior to the procedure.

- Renal insufficiency or solitary kidney is a contraindication in renal artery embolization, unless in potentially life-threatening situations.

Preprocedural Care

- Refer to Exhibit 19.1 for basic preprocedural care.

Anesthesia

- Procedure usually performed with moderate sedation and local anesthesia.

Intraprocedural Care

- Refer to Exhibit 19.2 for basic intraprocedural care.
- Patient placed on fluoroscopy table, usually in supine position.
- Heparin is usually mixed with normal saline on the sterile tray.
  - If patient is allergic to heparin, then alteplase might be used.

Postprocedural Care

- Refer to Exhibit 19.3 for basic postprocedural care.
- Arterial puncture site is observed for hematoma or bleeding prior to patient discharge for 2 hours if closure device is used (6 hours if manual compression is used).
  - Physician must be notified if hematoma or swelling occurs at the site.
- Bed rest is advised for 2 hours post femoral arterial puncture.
- If patient develops bleeding, then pressure should be applied at the access site and physician must be notified.
- Check distal pulses if embolization is performed in the extremities.
- Maintain pain control.

Follow-Up/Patient Education

- Patient follows up with primary care physician after procedure.
- Discharge instructions with contact information should be provided.

GASTROINTESTINAL BLEED

Introduction

- Acute gastrointestinal bleeding can be suspected to originate from the *upper gastrointestinal tract* when a patient presents with hematemesis and/or black tarry stools.

- Upper gastrointestinal bleeding is most commonly due to ulcers and rarely malignancy.
- If the bleeding is brisk, hypotension and tachycardia will be present, and resuscitative efforts will be essential.
- Diagnosis and treatment of the bleeding vessels are attempted first by gastroenterologist using an endoscope. If unsuccessful, interventional radiologist may be requested to localize and embolize the target vessel.
- For bleeding suspected to originate from the *lower gastrointestinal tract*, endoscopy is passed over for embolization techniques.
  - Embolization of the bleeding vessel is performed by gaining access to the femoral artery or left radial artery; an arterial sheath is placed to maintain access. A catheter is inserted into the sheath and advanced into the aorta while performing diagnostic angiograms.
  - The celiac trunk, superior mesenteric artery, or inferior mesenteric branches are investigated in detail because the target artery is usually a branch from one of these vessels. If a bleeding artery is found, it is packed with appropriately sized embolic coils until flow in the artery ceases.
  - Lower gastrointestinal bleeding is most commonly due to diverticulosis, an enterocolic vascular anomaly called angiodysplasia, or malignancy.

Indications

- Bleeding from the upper gastrointestinal tract that cannot be remedied with an endoscope
- Lower gastrointestinal tract bleeding

Contraindications

- No absolute contraindications when bleeding is life-threatening.
- Relative contraindications include renal insufficiency, contrast allergy, and untreatable coagulopathy.

Preprocedural Care

- Refer to Exhibit 19.1 for basic preprocedural care.
- Hypotensive patients should be fluid resuscitated prior to procedure, if acuity permits.

Anesthesia

- Embolization is performed under moderate sedation or general anesthesia.

Intraprocedural Care

- Refer to Exhibit 19.2 for basic intraprocedural care.
- Patient is placed in supine position.

Postprocedural Care

- Refer to Exhibit 19.3 for basic postprocedural care.
- Regular check of lower extremity pulses to assess for distal embolization.
- Vital sign trend demonstrating hypotension and/or tachycardia is suspect for ongoing hemorrhage.
- Patients may be placed on a PCA pump to control postprocedural pain.

Complications

- Nontarget embolization of the gut or other organs rarely leads to ischemia due to rich collateral supply in the abdomen.

Follow-Up/Patient Education

- Patient follows up with primary care physician after procedure.
- Discharge instructions with contact information should be provided.

Fast Facts

Bleeding localized to the upper gastrointestinal tract is best managed with initial endoscopic intervention, followed by transarterial embolization, if warranted. Bleeding localized to the lower intestinal tract may proceed straight to transarterial embolization after a preliminary abdominopelvic computed tomography angiography (CTA) or tagged red blood cells (RBC) scan in nuclear medicine.

25

Peripheral Arterial Disease and Hereditary Hemorrhagic Telangiectasia

Nana Ohene Baah and Ashwani Kumar Sharma

It is estimated that over 200 million people worldwide experience peripheral arterial disease (PAD), an occlusive disease that primarily affects the elderly. Symptoms range from no symptoms at all to those that severely affect a person's quality of life (claudication, pain, extremity weakness, nonhealing wounds, etc.). Those who smoke are at a higher risk of PAD.

Hereditary hemorrhagic telangiectasia (HHT), also referred to as Osler Weber Rendu syndrome (OWRS), is an autosomal dominant vascular proliferative disorder. Treatment can be performed in the interventional radiology suite.

In this chapter, you will discover:

1. Symptoms of peripheral artery disease
2. Treatment of peripheral artery disease
3. Hereditary hemorrhagic telangiectasia (HHT)
4. Treatment of pulmonary arteriovenous malformations (PAVMs) with embolotherapy

PERIPHERAL ARTERIAL DISEASE

Introduction

- Compromised blood flow to the extremities due to atherosclerotic calcifications of the feeding vessels.
- Symptoms develop when there is an imbalance between blood supply and demand.
  - Mild disease presents with reproducible discomfort and pain in a group of muscles upon exertion that resolves with rest.
  - Severe disease leads to pain even at rest and ischemic skin lesions, such as ulcerations.
- Treatment begins with lifestyle modifications and medical therapy before interventional therapies.
- Common minimally invasive revascularization techniques include angioplasty and stenting to improve flow to the distal extremity.
  - Access is gained to the femoral artery, and a sheath is placed into the femoral artery to maintain access. A catheter is inserted into the sheath and a runoff angiogram of the lower extremity is performed to determine areas of stenosis/occlusion. The area is then treated with balloon angioplasty or stent placement.

Indications

- Peripheral arterial disease refractory to lifestyle and medical management
- Critical limb ischemia

Contraindications

- Uncorrectable coagulopathy
- Allergy to metal in stent
- Allergy to contrast dye

Preprocedural Care

- Refer to Exhibit 19.1 for basic preprocedural care.

Anesthesia

- The procedure is performed with moderate sedation.

Intraprocedural Care

- Refer to Exhibit 19.2 for intraprocedural care.
- Place patient in supine position.
- Access site is usually the right femoral artery.

Postprocedural Care

- Refer to Exhibit 19.3 for postprocedural care.
- Regular checks of lower extremity pulses and ankle–brachial index are performed to assess for distal embolization.
- May be placed on a PCA pump to control postprocedure pain.

Complications

- May include emboli, pseudoaneurysm, or hematoma formation.
- Embolization of the atherosclerotic plaque presents with pain and diminished pulses distal to the site of intervention.
- Some patients may have a cool and painful foot with strong pulses.

Follow-Up/Patient Education

- Patient follows up with primary care physician after procedure.

Fast Facts

A tender pulsatile mass at the puncture site in the groin should prompt evaluation for a pseudoaneurysm.

HEREDITARY HEMORRHAGIC TELANGIECTASIA

Introduction

- HHT, also referred to as Osler Weber Rendu syndrome (OWRS), is an autosomal dominant vascular proliferative disorder. This hereditary disorder may present with an abnormal tangle of vessels in the nasal mucosa, oral mucosa, or on the skin. In the pulmonary system, this syndrome results in abnormal PAVMs, which create a direct connection between a pulmonary artery and a pulmonary vein without an intervening capillary bed.

- PAVMs can be asymptomatic yet lead to dyspnea, hemoptysis, brain infection, paradoxical embolization (arterial thrombosis), and high output heart failure.
- Embolization can be performed by interventional radiology to treat these malformations. The procedure utilizes ultrasound to access the right femoral vein or the right internal jugular vein. Fluoroscopy is then utilized for advancing a catheter through the right atrium, tricuspid valve, right ventricle and pulmonic valve, and into the pulmonary arteries. Pulmonary arterial and wedge pressure are performed to evaluate for the evidence of pulmonary arterial hypertension. A diagnostic pulmonary angiogram is performed to identify the vascular abnormality and for performing the embolization of the abnormality. Embolization is performed with coils or vascular plugs.

Indications

- PAVMs
- Pulmonary arteriovenous shunts
- Pulmonary artery aneurysms

Contraindications

- Contrast dye allergy
- Left bundle branch block

Preprocedural Care

- Refer to Exhibit 19.1 for basic preprocedural care.

Anesthesia

- Procedure usually performed with moderate sedation and local anesthesia.

Intraprocedural Care

- Refer to Exhibit 19.2 for basic intraprocedural care.
- Patient placed on fluoroscopy table, usually in supine position.
- Special attention should be paid to cardiac rhythm during wire or catheter advancement through the cardiac chambers because this can generate heart arrhythmia.
- Right femoral vein or right jugular vein is usually used for access.
- Prophylactic antibiotics, usually cefazolin 1 g IV.
- Heparin of 3,000 to 5,000 units is used with embolization.

Postprocedural Care

- Refer to Exhibit 19.3 for basic postprocedural care.
- Fever and chest pain are the most common side effects; these can occur several days after the procedure and are managed with nonsteroidal anti-inflammatory medications.

Complications

- Entry site hematoma
- Contrast-induced nephropathy
- Contrast reaction
- Paradoxical embolization
- Hemorrhage from the malformation

Follow-Up/Patient Education

- Advise patient to seek medical attention if having swelling at puncture site, persistent fevers or chills, or worsening hemoptysis.
- Patients with HHT may have multiple PAVMs that may be best managed with staged treatment sessions in 10- to 12-week intervals.
- Outpatient follow-up in 4 to 6 weeks.

Fast Facts

Prior EKG to evaluate and exclude a left bundle branch block is imperative. In patients with a left bundle branch block, transcutaneous pacing is advised in order to avoid a complete heart block during right cardiac catheterization.

26

Biliary Procedures

Ashwani Kumar Sharma

Percutaneous biliary procedures can be diagnostic or therapeutic, are performed under fluoroscopy, and allow for the visualization, evaluation, and possible treatment of the pathology.

In this chapter, you will discover:

1. The difference between diagnostic versus therapeutic biliary procedures
2. Common complications of biliary procedures
3. Biliary catheter care

PERCUTANEOUS TRANSHEPATIC CHOLANGIOGRAPHY

Introduction

- Percutaneous transhepatic cholangiography (PTC) is a diagnostic procedure performed under fluoroscopy and allows for the visualization and evaluation of the intrahepatic and extrahepatic bile ducts.
- PTC is performed by first puncturing the skin overlying the liver with a 21- or 22-gauge needle. Ultrasound is used to assess the anatomical structures and select a puncture site. The needle is advanced under fluoroscopic guidance using a contrast agent to visualize and access the biliary tract.

Indications

- Performed to evaluate the biliary system for dilatation, stenosis, or an obstruction

Contraindications

- Untreatable coagulopathy
- Recent antiplatelet agent use
- Relative contraindication includes large volume ascites

Preprocedural Care

- Refer to Exhibit 19.1 for basic preprocedural care.
- Prophylactic antibiotics are given.

Anesthesia

- Performed with moderate sedation

Intraprocedural Care

- Refer to Exhibit 19.2 for basic intraprocedural care.
- Place patient in supine position and prep the right upper quadrant of the abdomen.

Postprocedural Care

- Refer to Exhibit 19.3 for basic postprocedural care.

Complications

- Subcapsular hematoma or peritoneal bleeding
  - Monitor for discomfort, hypotension, and tachycardia.
- Peritonitis may develop from a bile leak.
  - Monitor for abdominal pain, tenderness, and guarding.

Follow-Up/Patient Education

- Patient follows up with primary care physician after procedure.

PERCUTANEOUS BILIARY DRAINAGE

Introduction

- A therapeutic procedure performed to drain bile from the biliary system.
- The first part of the procedure is identical to a percutaneous transhepatic cholangiogram. After access is gained and a cholangiogram is performed, a wire is passed into the needle and guided into the bile ducts under fluoroscopy. A locking pigtail catheter is placed with the tip curled in the duodenum. The catheter is sutured to the skin, a drainage bag is connected, and dressings are applied.

Indications

- This procedure allows for the removal of bile in cases of obstruction, biliary infection, and bile leaks.

Contraindications

- No absolute contraindications.
- Relative contraindications include untreatable coagulopathy, recent antiplatelet agent use, and large volume ascites.

Preprocedural Care

- Refer to Exhibit 19.1 for basic preprocedural care.
- Prophylactic antibiotics are given.
- Ultrasound is used to evaluate liver and determine access site.

Anesthesia

- Percutaneous biliary drainage is performed with moderate sedation.

Intraprocedural Care

- Refer to Exhibit 19.2 for basic intraprocedural care.
- Place patient in supine position and prep the right upper quadrant of the abdomen.

Postprocedural Care

- Refer to Exhibit 19.3 for basic postprocedural care.
- Dressing changes should be performed daily.
- Drainage from the catheter should be recorded every 8 hours.

Complications

- Monitor for leakage around the catheter, signs of infection at the skin site, or a significant change in output occurs (notify physician).
- Sepsis, although rare, can occur from the procedure.
    - Monitor for change in vital signs (increasing temperature and heart rate, decreasing blood pressure) and notify physician.
- As with a PTC, patients can develop a subcapsular hematoma, peritoneal bleeding, or peritonitis from a bile leak.

Follow-Up/Patient Education

- Catheter is removed by a radiologist when the primary care physician considers it appropriate.
- Patient should contact primary care physician if puncture site demonstrates signs of infection.

Fast Facts

The catheter should be flushed with 10 mL of normal saline if drainage stops or flushed daily if the catheter is capped.

PERCUTANEOUS CHOLECYSTOSTOMY

Introduction

- Percutaneous cholecystostomy is a therapeutic procedure that drains the gallbladder by placing a catheter into its lumen.
- Ultrasound is used to assess the anatomy and select a puncture site in the right upper abdomen. The gallbladder is accessed using a trocar catheter or a sheathed needle. A floppy wire is passed through the needle into the gallbladder. A tract is created, and a locking pigtail catheter is placed with the tip curled in the gallbladder. Bile fluid samples are removed for gram stain and culture.

Indications

- Typically performed in acute patients who are poor surgical candidates

Contraindications

- No absolute contraindications.
- Relative contraindications include untreatable coagulopathy, recent antiplatelet agent use, and large volume ascites.

Preprocedural Care

- Refer to Exhibit 19.1 for basic preprocedural care.
- Prophylactic antibiotics are given.

Anesthesia

- Performed with moderate sedation

Intraprocedural Care

- Refer to Exhibit 19.2 for basic intraprocedural care.
- Place patient in supine position and prep the right upper quadrant of the abdomen.

Postprocedural Care

- Refer to Exhibit 19.3 for basic postprocedural care.
- Dressing changes should be performed daily.
- Drainage from the catheter should be recorded every 8 hours.

Complications

- Monitor for leakage around the catheter, signs of infection at the skin site, or a significant change in output (notify physician).
- Major complications include bile leak leading to peritonitis, bleeding, and sepsis.

Follow-Up/Patient Education

- Catheter is removed by a radiologist when the primary care physician considers it appropriate.
- Patient should contact primary care physician if puncture site demonstrates signs of infection.

Flush the catheter with 10 mL of normal saline every 6 to 8 hours or if drainage stops.

27

Percutaneous Procedures
Ashwani Kumar Sharma

Procedures performed in an interventional radiology suite have a number of benefits for the patient, including shortened procedural time (pre, intra, and post), improved patient comfort, less procedural risk, and often being more affordable. The use of image guidance assists the interventional radiologist in heightened accuracy of the procedure, as the direct path of the procedure can usually be determined before the procedure even begins.

In this chapter, you will discover:

1. How an abscess is drained
2. The process to biopsy tissue
3. Indication for a nephrostomy tube placement

ABSCESS DRAINAGE

Introduction

- Percutaneous technique used for abscess drainage offers many advantages to traditional open surgical drainage and has become the first-line therapy in treating infected fluid collections.

- If the abscess is located superficially, the procedure is straightforward.
  - Deeper locations can present a challenge due to increased risk for injury to the surrounding structures.
- The procedure can be performed under ultrasound, CT, or fluoroscopic guidance.
  - The most appropriate modality and optimal tract to the collection is determined by the location and nature of the collection.
- Small collections are aspirated, and the collected samples are sent to the lab for analysis. Frequently ordered tests include gram stain and culture.
- Larger collections are accessed with a needle followed by creation of a tract and placement of a locking pigtail catheter, which is then sutured to the skin and attached to a drainage bag with a three-way stopcock.

Indications

- Percutaneous abscess drainage can be diagnostic and/or therapeutic.

Contraindications

- No absolute contraindications

Preprocedural Care

- Refer to Exhibit 19.1 for basic preprocedural care.
- Give prophylactic antibiotics to prevent infection if deemed necessary by physician.

Anesthesia

- Local anesthesia for small collections and moderate sedation for larger collections

Intraprocedural Care

- Refer to Exhibit 19.2 for basic intraprocedural care.
- Patient is positioned on the procedural table in a variety of positions depending on the characteristics of the collection. The position is determined by the physician.

Postprocedural Care

- Refer to Exhibit 19.3 for basic postprocedural care.
- Record drainage from the catheter every 8 hours.
- Decrease drainage daily and remove the catheter when less than 20 mL per day of fluid is returned.
- Poor output or occlusion of the catheter can be remedied with tissue plasminogen activator (tPA) infusion.

Complications

- Hemorrhage, sepsis, and peritonitis.
- If there is an increase in fluid drainage, especially greater than 50 mL of fluid per day, the patient might have developed a fistula. Notify the physician.

Follow-Up/Patient Education

- Catheter is removed by a radiologist when the primary care physician considers it appropriate.
- Patient should contact primary care physician if puncture site demonstrates signs of infection.

Fast Facts

When a drainage catheter is placed, the catheter should be flushed toward the collection and toward the drainage bag with 10 mL of normal saline every 8 hours to prevent occlusion.

PERCUTANEOUS BIOPSY

Description

- One of the most common procedures performed by interventional radiologists.
- A tissue sample from the target lesion can differentiate a benign from malignant process and identify the type of benign or malignant process occurring.
- Common structures biopsied percutaneously include the thyroid, superficial skin and muscle structures, lungs, abdominal organs, pelvic organs, lymph nodes, and bone.

- The type of imaging modality (ultrasound, fluoroscopy, CT, or MRI) will depend on the type and location of the target lesion.
- Percutaneous biopsies can be performed with a variety of needles depending on the location and the type of lesion suspected. After access is gained to the target tissue, several passes are made to ensure an adequate sample is taken. The sample is placed in a formalin container and sent to the pathology department.

Indication

- Percutaneous biopsies are performed to sample tissue.

Contraindication

- No absolute contraindications.
- Relative contraindication includes uncorrectable coagulopathy.

Preprocedural Care

- Refer to Exhibit 19.1 for basic preprocedural care.

Anesthesia

- Percutaneous biopsies are performed with local anesthesia; conscious sedation can be used if necessary.

Intraprocedural Care

- Refer to Exhibit 19.2 for basic intraprocedural care.

Postprocedural Care

- Refer to Exhibit 19.3 for basic postprocedural care.

Complications

- The most common, although rare, complications are bleeding and infection.

Follow-Up/Patient Education

- Patient follows up with primary care physician after procedure.
- Patients should contact primary care physician if puncture site demonstrates signs of infection

PERCUTANEOUS NEPHROSTOMY TUBE PLACEMENT

Introduction

- Drain the upper urinary tract in cases of acute or chronic obstructive uropathy.
- Patients can develop a urinary tract obstruction for various reasons from stones to tumors, and timely placement of a nephrostomy tube can prove essential in maintaining renal function and preventing urosepsis.
- During tube placement, ultrasound is used to assess the anatomy and select the optimal approach to the kidney. The renal collecting system is accessed with a puncture needle, a wire is fed through the needle, and a tract is created for placement of a locking pigtail catheter. The catheter tip is curled in the renal pelvis and the free end is sutured to the skin.
- Other indication for a percutaneous nephrostomy tube includes access to the urinary tract for interventions and to divert urine in cases of a urine leak or urinoma.

Indications

- Obstructive uropathy
- Urinary diversion
- Percutaneous access for interventions
- Pyonephrosis

Contraindications

- Untreatable coagulopathy

Preprocedural Care

- Refer to Exhibit 19.1 for basic preprocedural care.

Anesthesia

- Percutaneous nephrostomy tube placement is performed with moderate sedation.

Intraprocedural Care

- Refer to Exhibit 19.2 for basic intraprocedural care.
- Place patient in prone position.
- Administer prophylactic antibiotics.

Postprocedural Care

- Refer to Exhibit 19.3 for basic postprocedural care.
- Record fluid intake and urine output. Blood-tinged urine can occur for the first 48 hours post procedure, but frank hematuria should not be present.
- Flush the catheter every 4 hours with 5 mL of normal saline if clots are present (must have a physician's order to flush a nephrostomy tube).

Complications

- Major complications from the procedure include massive hemorrhage, injury to surrounding organs, or sepsis.
  - Patients with hemorrhage can present with hypotension and may require surgery or embolization to control the bleeding.
- Minor complications include a urine leak and pain at the procedure site.

Follow Up/Patient Education

- Catheter is removed by a radiologist when the primary care physician considers it appropriate.
- Patient should contact primary care physician if puncture site demonstrates signs of infection.

28

Filters and Foreign Bodies

Ashwani Kumar Sharma

In this chapter, you will discover:

1. Process to retrieve foreign bodies utilizing interventional radiology (IR) services
2. Indications for inferior vena cava (IVC) filter placement
3. Types of IVC filters available

VENA CAVA FILTERS

Introduction

- These devices are usually placed in the inferior vena cava to prevent pulmonary embolism by trapping thrombus that can break from lower extremity thrombi or placed in the superior vena cava for patients with upper extremity deep venous thrombus (DVT).
- Pulmonary embolism or DVT is usually treated pharmacologically with anticoagulation therapy. Vena cava filters are employed in cases where there is a contraindication for pharmacological treatment such as bleeding, in cases of failed anticoagulation therapy, or in cases of large clot burden.
- These filters can also be used prophylactically in patients with high risk for developing DVT, such as trauma or surgical patients who will be immobilized for an extensive length of time.

- There are three main categories of filters:
    - Permanent filters are placed permanently and are not intended to be removed or repositioned.
    - Optional filters are designed so that they can be retrieved, if desired.
    - Temporary filters have to be removed.
- Optional and temporary filters are more commonly used, and the Society of Interventional Radiology recommends removal of these filters.
- Different manufacturer types of these filters exist, and they vary by design and delivery system, including vein for access.

Indications

- Documented DVT or high risk for developing DVT with inability to properly treat with pharmacological therapy.

Contraindications

- Total thrombosis of the vena cava
- Lack of access or imaging for delivery of the filter
- Allergy to filter components
- Bacteremia

Preprocedural Care

- Refer to Exhibit 19.1 for basic preprocedural care.

Anesthesia

- Procedure is usually performed with moderate sedation and local anesthesia.

Intraprocedural Care

- Refer to Exhibit 19.2 for basic intraprocedural care.
- Place patient on fluoroscopy table, usually in supine position.
- Ultrasound may be used for identifying the venous site initially, and then fluoroscopy.
- Venous access for placement of filter can be the common femoral veins or the jugular veins. A direct approach into the SVC can also be performed.
- Venography is performed during the exam to assess for proper placement of filter.

Postprocedural Care

- Refer to Exhibit 19.3 for basic postprocedural care.
- Assess lower extremities for increased swelling, which can indicate clotting of IVC filter.

Complications

- Contrast reaction
- Contrast-induced nephropathy
- Entry site hematoma
- Infection
- Lower extremity edema
- Recurrent pulmonary embolism
- Cava thrombosis
- Filter migration, fracture, or failure

Fast Facts

Be sure that the patient receives product information, including name of product, model, and lot number of the filter placed. They may need this information in the future when having an MRI, if there is a product recall from the company, or if complications occur.

Follow-Up/Patient Education

- Outpatient follow-up in 4 to 6 weeks.
- Retrievable filters: Schedule venous doppler ultrasound to assess for remaining venous thrombus prior to filter removal. Follow-up appointment for removal of the filter is determined by the patient's need for the filter and the manufacturer's recommendation for retrieval.
- Permanent filters: Abdominal radiographs are taken every 3 to 4 years to evaluate filter position and integrity.

VENA CAVA FILTER RETRIEVAL

Introduction

- The new types of vena cava filters are designed to be removed. Removal is recommended and reduces the risk of filter-related complications.

- Access is obtained into a large vein, such as the internal jugular vein or femoral vein, depending on the filter design. Cavogram is performed by advancing a catheter and injecting contrast to visualize the vena cava. Sheath and snare are utilized to remove the filter.
- Imaging demonstrating resolution of previous DVT is usually performed.

Indications

- Filter is no longer needed due to adequate venous thrombus therapy.
- Patient is no longer at a risk for venous thrombus embolus.
- Filter fails to offer protection against venous thrombus embolus due to structural failure or filter migration.
- Filter causing pain.

Contraindications

- Persistent DVT or retained thrombus within the filter.
- Patient remains high risk for venous thrombus embolism.
- Lack of venous access for filter retrieval.
- Terminal illness with less than 6-month life expectancy.

Preprocedural Care

- Refer to Exhibit 19.1 for basic preprocedural care.

Anesthesia

- Procedure usually performed with moderate sedation and local anesthesia.

Intraprocedural Care

- Refer to Exhibit 19.2 for basic intraprocedural care.
- Place patient on fluoroscopy table, usually in supine position.
- Ultrasound may be used for identifying the venous site initially, and then fluoroscopy is utilized.

Postprocedural Care

- Refer to Exhibit 19.3 for basic postprocedural care.

Complications

- Contrast reaction
- Contrast-induced nephropathy
- Infection
- Pain at the access site

Follow-Up/Patient Education

- Patient follows up with primary care physician after procedure.
- Therapy and prophylaxis for venous thrombosis can be resumed and continued until no longer clinically needed.

FOREIGN BODY RETRIEVAL

Description

- Foreign bodies can be dislodged, and it may be necessary to remove them.
    - Such scenarios include broken intravascular catheters, wires, nonvascular catheters, stents, or other foreign bodies.
- Procedure for removal of these foreign bodies depends on the location and the type of foreign body.
- Snares, forceps, and other instruments can be utilized to remove these bodies.
- Imaging demonstrating these foreign bodies is usually performed prior to the procedure.

Indications

- Foreign body posing a significant risk to the patient

Contraindications

- Case dependent

Preprocedural Care

- Refer to Exhibit 19.1 for basic preprocedural care.

Anesthesia

- Procedure can be performed with moderate sedation or minimal sedation.

Intraprocedural Care

■ Refer to Exhibit 19.2 for basic intraprocedural care.

Fast Facts

Ensure foreign body is removed in its entirety, especially if it breaks during the procedure.

Postprocedural Care

■ Refer to Exhibit 19.3 for basic postprocedural care.

Complications

■ Infection, bleeding, and injury to the organs surrounding the foreign body

Follow-Up/Patient Education

■ Patient follows up with primary care physician after procedure.
■ Patient should contact primary care physician if puncture site demonstrates signs of infection or if having swelling at puncture site, fevers, or chills.

V

Diagnostic and Other Imaging Modalities

29

X-Ray, Mammography, Nuclear Medicine, Ultrasound

Valerie Aarne Grossman

All areas of the imaging environment pose a different set of challenges and expectations for the radiology nurse. Interventional radiology, CT scan, and MRI scan are the areas that utilize nursing personnel to the greatest degree; however, there are many other modalities within radiology that may also need the expertise of a nurse. The nurse who practices in a radiology setting must be ready to change direction at a moment's notice. Infinite reasons exist that may necessitate a radiologist, radiologic technologist, or a patient to call for a nurse.

In this chapter, you will discover:

1. Patient preparation for exams
2. Necessary patient screening
3. Differences in imaging technology

PROJECTION RADIOGRAPHY "X-RAY"

The use of radiation to capture images was first discovered (by accident) in 1895 by Wilhelm Roentgen, a German physics professor. He experimented on his wife and first presented his discovery in 1896;

the same year, it was first used on patients in a clinical setting. The use of film and chemicals to develop the x-ray images has now been replaced by a digital process and computer screen. "Plain x-rays" remain the first-line image for many patient care situations.

In some countries, nurses with additional training are permitted to order x-rays for patients (Thompson, Murphy, Robinson, & Buckley, 2016). In the United States, each state establishes the scope of practice for healthcare providers and decides who can order x-rays.

Fluoroscopy

This is a special application of x-ray imaging where real-time imaging occurs to track motion. At times, contrast may be used to augment the image in the form of oral, rectal, cavity, or intravenous contrast dye. The contrast will absorb the x-rays, highlight the motion process, and capture the images. This process is useful in assessing digestive tract peristalsis or blood flow through vessels.

Nursing interventions in this modality are often minimal to nothing at all. Radiologists and radiologic technologists provide the care for patients in this area.

MAMMOGRAPHY

This low-dose radiographic technique has been practiced for more than 50 years to discover breast cysts or tumors. A *screening mammogram* looks for breast disease in asymptomatic women while *diagnostic mammogram* diagnoses breast disease in symptomatic women or those with a finding during a screening mammogram. This new technology has many positive influences for both patients and staff that include the following:

- Easier for the patient
  - Decreased need for additional images or return trips for additional films
- Decreased amount of staff time to obtain/process images
- Increased interpretation accuracy of the radiologist
  - Easy identification of dense versus nondense breast tissue and manipulation of images for more accurate interpretations

Nursing care in the mammography suite is minimal as the images are obtained by a radiologic technologist. Nurses may be utilized during adverse events or biopsy procedures.

Patient Screening

The following indications for mammography should be considered:

- Annual exams for asymptomatic women aged 45 and older at average risk for breast cancer
- Women under age 40 at increased risk for breast cancer
  - Known mutation or genetic syndrome with increased breast cancer risk starting annually between ages 25 and 30
    - BRCA1 or BRCA2 mutation gene carriers
  - First-degree relative with known BRCA mutation, starting annually between ages 25 and 30
  - Sisters or mothers with premenopausal breast cancer, starting annually between the ages of 25 and 30 or 10 years earlier than the age of relative's diagnosis
  - History of chest (mantle) radiation received between the ages of 10 and 30, starting annually and 8 years after the radiation therapy, but not before age 25
  - Biopsy-proven lobular neoplasia, atypical ductal hyperplasia (ADH), ductal carcinoma in-situ (DCIS), invasive breast cancer, or ovarian cancer: starting annually from the time of diagnosis regardless of age (ACR, 2013)
- Woman with breast augmentation
  - Must receive mammography services from a center equipped to image breasts with implants (Lee et al., 2010)

Fast Facts

Proper patient preparation is essential to ensure a quality patient experience and perfection in the image quality of the exam. Where possible, call the patient prior to the scheduled visit, answer their questions, and explain what they should expect while in your care. When the patient arrives, welcome them warmly and help to calm any concerns they may have.

Patient Education for Mammography

Patient education should begin when the appointment is first scheduled. The patient should be advised in following appropriate organizational preparation (i.e., insurance card, photo identification, avoiding wearing deodorant/power/creams, etc.). The mammography technologist will continue the education by explaining the imaging procedure to the patient, answering her questions, helping to reduce the patient's anxiety, and instructing how the results will be handled.

NUCLEAR MEDICINE

Images are obtained by injecting the patient with a radiopharmaceutical that locates to a particular type of body organ or tissue type and is then imaged with a gamma camera. Different from other imaging modalities, the radiation comes from inside of the patient's body to the outside, where a camera obtains the image (other modalities direct the radiation from the camera through the body to obtain images). The most common images are obtained of the:

- Brain
- Heart, lungs
- Thyroid, parathyroid
- Bone
- Liver, gallbladder, spleen, or kidney
- Vessels causing internal bleeding
- Infection
- Collection of cells

Positron emission tomography (PET) is another imaging technique used in nuclear medicine, where a radioactive, biological substance is injected into the patient and localizes to metabolically active tissues such as a cancerous area (SNMMI, 2013).

A nurse may be called to this area to perform point-of-care testing (POCT) glucose, place an intravenous (IV), inject certain medication that may be used for scans, or respond to adverse patient events.

Patient Screening

Patients will be screened for a medical history including allergies and pregnancy status.

Fast Facts

Some patients will receive radioactive contrast and may need special documentation if they plan to travel through security checkpoints such as at an airport. Where possible, call the patient prior to the scheduled visit, explain what they should expect, and ask if they will need this special documentation post exam.

Patient Education for Nuclear Medicine

Patient education should begin when the appointment is first scheduled. The patient should be advised per organizational preparation policy (i.e., insurance card, photo identification, wearing comfortable clothing, nothing by mouth [NPO] for certain exams, etc.). Upon the patient's arrival to the department, the nuclear medicine technologist will continue the educational process by explaining the imaging procedure, answering questions, and providing instruction regarding how test results can be obtained. This additional education helps to reduce the patient's anxiety.

ULTRASOUND

This imaging technique uses high-frequency sound waves to create the image that is interpreted by the radiologist. The first use of ultrasound occurred in the 1940s and has grown in use since then.

- Ultrasound scan refers to the "procedure" of obtaining images.
  - External: probe placed outside of the body, looking inward
  - Internal: probe placed inside the body
    - Vaginal internal probe to look at uterus and ovaries (women)
    - Rectal internal probe to look at the prostate gland (males)
  - Endoscopic: probe placed through the mouth into the esophagus
    - Evaluates the esophagus, chest lymph nodes, or the stomach
- Sonogram is the actual image produced.
- Doppler ultrasound images movement (i.e., blood flowing through a vessel).
  - Color may be used to identify flow patterns.
- Ultrasound is useful in diagnostic imaging of the organs, including:
  - Eye
  - Chest: heart, vessels, lungs (images poorly through air; however, helpful when identifying fluid collection in the lungs)
  - Abdomen: stomach, liver
  - Musculoskeletal: tendons, muscles, joints
  - Genitourinary/obstetrical: scrotum, uterus
  - Vascular: blood vessels
- Therapeutic ultrasound is the use of sound waves to:
  - Cause coagulation necrosis of tissue
  - Stimulate bone growth
  - Help drugs pass the bloodbrain barrier

- Phacoemulsification of cataracts
- Lithotripsy of kidney stones
- POCT ultrasound is a useful "beside tool" in areas from the ED to the anesthesia department, finding its way to assist with patient assessment to initiation of care (i.e., IV line placement, bladder scanners, Dopplers, etc.).

For routine ultrasound exams, little nursing care is required. However, a nurse utilizing ultrasound to assist with IV cannulation must have already undergone special training. Additionally, if ultrasound is used during a procedure with a physician, the nurse may administer pain medications and/or moderate sedation (see Chapter 7, Sedation and Monitoring).

Patient Screening

Ultrasound technology is highly dependent on the skill of the person using the equipment as well as the body habitus of the patient being examined (i.e., high-quality images are difficult to obtain on very thin or obese patients). Minimal patient screening or preparation is needed prior to the use of ultrasound.

Patient Education for Ultrasound

Patient education should begin when the appointment is first scheduled. The patient should be advised per organizational preparation policy (i.e., insurance card, photo identification, wearing comfortable clothing, NPO for certain exams, full bladder for other exams, etc.). The person performing the POCT ultrasound or the sonographer will continue the educational process by explaining the imaging procedure to the patient, answering questions, helping to reduce the patient's anxiety, and instructing how the results will be handled.

References

American College of Radiology. (2013). *ACR practice guideline for the performance of screening and diagnostic mammography*. Retrieved from https://www.acr.org/-/media/ACR/Files/Practice-Parameters/Screen-Diag-Mammo.pdf

Lee, C. H., Dershaw, D. D., Kopans, D., Evans, P., Monsees, B., Monticciolo, D., & Burhenne, L. W.(2010). Breast cancer screening with imaging: Recommendations from the Society of Breast Imaging and the ACR on the use of mammography, breast MRI, breast ultrasound, and other technologies for the detection of clinically occult breast cancer. *Journal of the American College of Radiology, 7*, 18–27. doi:10.1016/j.jacr.2009.09.022

Society of Nuclear Medicine and Molecular Imaging. (2013). *Practice guidelines.* Retrieved from https://www.guidelinecentral.com/summaries/organizations/society-of-nuclear-medicine-and-molecular-imaging-snmmi/

Thompson, N., Murphy, M., Robinson, J., & Buckley, T. (2016). Improving nurse initiated X-ray practice through action research. *Journal of Medical Radiation Sciences, 63*(4), 203–208. doi:10.1002/jmrs.197

VI

Special Issues in
Radiology Nursing

30

Fragile and High-Risk Populations

Valerie Aarne Grossman

The radiology environment is diverse and changes quickly. The radiology nurse often does not know what is going to happen in the next few minutes: The variability of the patient population leaves a great deal of unknown factors that are unable to be planned for. Each patient brings unique identifiers that may add challenges to the nurse's goal of providing patient- and family-focused imaging care. The nurse must recognize the unique needs of each individual patient and work to meet those needs with the ultimate outcome of safe, quality patient care.

In this chapter, you will discover:

1. The care of a pediatric patient
2. The care of a geriatric patient
3. Techniques in the care of high-risk/fragile patients

Radiology nursing is an exciting arena: The variability of the patient population leaves a great deal of unknown factors that are unable to be planned for.

PEDIATRIC

- The better the cooperation of the patient, the better the image being obtained.

- Educate the child (and guardian) prior to entering the modality, if possible.
  - Use simple terms, just the basics, do not scare the child (or parent!)
  - Advise of big room, fancy camera, funny smells, weird noises, and the like.
- Never leave the child unattended.
- When possible, allow parent to remain in the room with the child.
- Allow child to bring a comfort item (toy, blanket, etc.).
- At times, sedation or immobilization (Velcro, blankets, etc.) may be utilized.
- Use distraction when appropriate (visual, audio, personal interactions, etc.).
- Demonstrate using parent ("Daddy is going to lie on the table first, then it's your turn.")
- Protect the child from radiation exposure as much as is possible (Linder & Schiska, 2007; Matich, 2011; Munn & Jordan, 2013; Reilly, Byrne, & Ely, 2012).

Fast Facts

Take the extra time to include the patent/caregiver in the care of the child as this will help the child to be more comfortable in the radiology setting—an environment that can be quite scary to a child. Make the exam seem like "play"; where possible, allow the child's comfort item to be close to them. This will promote a successful exam and decrease the potential for a traumatic experience for the child.

GERIATRIC

- Identify communication barriers (hearing impaired, slow speech pattern, slow cognition, etc.) and physical barriers (decreased strength, slower walking, unsteady gait, easily fatigued, diminished eyesight, etc.), and find solutions.
- Carefully assess patient's history, current medications, and so forth.
- Watch for fragility (easy skin tearing, difficult IV cannulation, easy bruising).
- Foster autonomy wherever possible, communicate on their level.
- Provide for physical comfort (padding, wedges, blankets, etc.).

CHEMICALLY ALTERED

- Patients who have received pain medication or sedation prior to coming to radiology may easily fall, have decreased ability to cooperate with directions, may easily forget instructions, and so forth.
- Patients who have consumed mind-altering chemicals may be uncooperative and, at times, are a danger to the radiology staff. Monitor them closely; utilize security if necessary.

MORBIDLY OBESE

- Be open, honest, and nonjudgmental with larger patients if there are concerns regarding their care due to their size.
- Provide appropriate-sized patient gown, maintain privacy and dignity for patient.
- Obtain current and accurate weight on patient; do not use their stated weight.
- Verify table weight limit prior to placing patient on the table.
- Educate patient regarding the use of wedges, belts, and other safety devices to maintain proper patient position during exam.
- Contrast may be weight based: Be careful of dose limits.
- Measure patient girth to be sure patient will fit in scanner gantries/apertures.

COGNITIVE DISORDERS

- Identify the ability of the patient to comprehend instructions.
- Speak at a level that is understood by the patient/family.

EXTREME STRESS OR FEAR

- Imperative for staff to recognize the anxiety level of the patient.
- Work to provide a confident and calm environment for the patient/family.
- Fear of the unknown is powerful, so work to educate the patient from the very first interaction.

Be open and honest in all communication. Do not judge the patient, their beliefs, or their personal lifestyle choices. Accept them, welcome them, and help them to be comfortable in the radiology setting.

CULTURALLY DIVERSE

- Different groups may perceive a situation differently.
  - You may not understand the background of each patient. However, be sensitive to the fears a patient may have from not understanding the technical radiology setting.
- Work to find a common ground of understanding: Use interpreters, listen for concerns, take time to teach and answer questions, provide for patient comfort, and so forth.
- Portray confidence, acceptance, patience, and friendliness to all patients.
- Identify own bias or prejudice, work to keep them out of the workplace (Grossman, 2003; Jan & Nardi, 2005).

References

Grossman, V. (2003). Cross cultural empathy. In *Quick reference to triage*. Philadelphia, PA: Lippincott, Williams, & Wilkins.

Jan, S., & Nardi, D. (2005). Radiology nursing and the Asian population. *Journal of Radiology Nursing, 24*(4), 79–84.

Linder, J., & Schiska, A (2007). Imaging children: Tips and tricks. *Journal of Radiology Nursing, 26*(1), 23–25. doi:10.1016/j.jradnu.2007.01.007

Matich, S. (2011). Just pediatrics: Radiation and the pediatric patient. *Journal of Radiology Nursing, 30*(4), 170–171. doi:10.1016/j.jradnu.2011.08.003

Munn, Z., & Jordan, Z. (2013). Interventions to reduce anxiety, distress, and the need for sedation in pediatric patients undergoing magnetic resonance imaging: A systematic review. *Journal of Radiology Nursing, 32*(2), 87–96.

Reilly, L., Byrne, A., & Ely, E. (2012). Does the use of an immobilizer provide a quality MR image of the brain in infants? *Journal of Radiology Nursing, 31*(3), 91–96. doi:10.1016/j.jradnu.2012.04.002

31

Communication Essentials Between the ED and Radiology

Anna C. Montejano and Lynn Sayre Visser

The Joint Commission's National Safety Goals discuss hand-off communication as a necessary standard identified in 2010 as a hospital requirement. Poor hand-off communication between the sender and receiver can result in a delay of care or, even worse, a sentinel event. Each organization makes decisions on a method that works to ensure effective communication to improve patient safety (The Joint Commission, 2017). The collaboration between the ED and the radiology department is a critical part of this process.

In this chapter, you will discover:

1. Two reasons why effective communication between the ED and the radiology department is important
2. How a "ticket to ride" can improve ineffective communication
3. Two reasons for a delay in turnaround time between the ED and radiology

INEFFECTIVE COMMUNICATION

Ineffective communication may result in the following:

- Patients may sustain an injury due to a "fall risk."
- Delay in transportation to the radiology department due to unavailability of staff or the medical provider needed for a procedure, lack of room availability, or the ED staff is in the process of initiating care, stabilizing the patient, and so forth.
- Patient does not understand why there is a delay in their care.
- Radiology staff exposed to an infectious disease.
- Delay in performing a radiologic exam due to the patient's weight exceeding the weight limit of certain radiological equipment, such as the CT scanner.

WHEN RADIOLOGY IS READY FOR THE ED PATIENT

Both radiology and the ED are dynamic environments. Coordination of schedules must occur to optimize a smooth process in the care of patients. Clear communication between the radiology and ED staff, prior to the patient being transported from the ED to radiology, enhances departmental efficiency, patient outcomes, and improves patient satisfaction.

PREPARING THE ED PATIENT FOR RADIOLOGY

The ED nurse should be informed prior to the patient being transported to radiology for the following reasons:

- Certain diagnostic tests may require the completion of a questionnaire prior to patient transport. One example is the required screening documentation before the patient can undergo an MRI.
- Some patients may require portable oxygen during transport. Prioritize ensuring the oxygen tank is available, full, and with the patient.

Fast Facts

Be sure the oxygen tank used for transport has enough oxygen to support the needs of the patient. A higher flow may require a full

PART VI   SPECIAL ISSUES IN RADIOLOGY NURSING

242

tank while a lower flow rate may only require a minimum of 500 psi (pounds per square inch). Remember to bring enough oxygen in the event there is a delay in radiology. Be proactive! Make sure there is a sufficient amount of oxygen!

- Diagnostic results, such as a glomerular filtration rate (GFR) or EKG, may be required prior to a radiologic procedure.
- Intravenous (IV) access may be required: Ensure the catheter size and placement location are appropriate for the procedure ordered. If the patient has a central line, such as a mediport, confirm with radiology if this catheter can be used for high-pressure contrast administration.
- If the patient is receiving IV fluid, the nurse may need to slow down the rate or hang a new IV bag prior to transport to prevent the IV bag from becoming empty.
- The patient may require medication prior to transport to control anxiety, provide pain relief, and/or begin IV antibiotics to fight an infection.
- If the ED is waiting for a urine sample from the patient, this information should be communicated to the radiology staff so that a potential specimen will not be discarded.
- Valuables, including jewelry (do not forget the ones that are not visible), may need to be removed prior to obtaining films. Do not forget about items that contain metal, such as bras with underwire!
- Acutely ill patients may require a nurse to accompany them to radiology to closely monitor for any changes that may result in decompensation.

Fast Facts

ED patients often require a multitude of orders that must be carried out in addition to the radiology test. ED staff must prioritize the needed tests and communicate clearly to the radiology staff as to when the patient is ready to be transported.

UPON TRANSPORT TO RADIOLOGY—TICKET TO RIDE

The Joint Commission's International Patient Safety Goal #2 focuses on enhancing communication (World Health Organization, 2007).

Between 1995 and 2006, reports to The Joint Commission confirmed insufficient communication as the primary cause of sentinel events (Joint Commission Center for Transforming Healthcare, 2013). As a result of these reports, the Ticket to Ride was developed as one avenue for standardizing communication among staff and supports to improve patient safety. Depending on the organization's process, there may be a combination of paper and electronic methods for this communication process.

Components of Ticket to Ride should include the following:

- Placing the Ticket to Ride on colored paper for easy visualization.
- Developing the tool in a situation/background/assessment/recommendation (SBAR) format to ensure a thorough and standardized form of communication (World Health Organization, 2007).
  - *Situation* includes the imaging studies ordered for the patient (e.g., CT) and the reason for the procedure (e.g., chest x-ray to rule out pneumonia). Verifying that the patient is wearing an identification bracelet with an accurate date of birth and correct spelling of their name is critical!
  - *Background* provides information regarding the patient's diagnosis, code status, and orientation. Additionally, fall risk, ability to stand, isolation, communication (native language), DNR status, and deficits in hearing or vision are identified.
  - *Assessment* includes the patient's current condition. Invaluable information to report to transporting staff includes the presence of IV lines, tubes or drains, oxygen needs, or sedating medications given.
  - *Recommendation* includes providing a phone number in the ED to call for questions as well as the patient's primary nurse/physician.

PATIENT RETURNING TO THE ED FROM RADIOLOGY

The ED nurse should be informed when the patient returns to the ED. This practice will allow:

- Verbal patient hand-off, which supports best practice
- The nurse to anticipate radiology report results
- Oxygen therapy to be continued by preventing the oxygen tank from becoming empty resulting in an unsafe situation
- Cardiac monitoring to be resumed per provider's order

- Provider's orders, which were not initiated prior to transport, or prompt initiation of postprocedure orders, such as the need for a thrombolytic for a newly diagnosed ischemic stroke
- Monitoring the patient for any adverse reaction to medications received, such as contrast

Fast Facts

Communication with the ED nurse that the patient has returned to the ED supports best practice in patient hand-off, enhancing patient safety and yielding opportunity for the delivery of timely continued care.

SITUATIONS THAT MAY DELAY RADIOLOGY TURNAROUND TIME

A number of reasons require the ED staff to delay patient transport to radiology. Likewise, the radiology staff may need to delay accepting the ED patient. Both the ED and radiology staff must continuously prioritize care of their patients.

Reasons for delay prior to transport to of the ED patient to radiology may include:

- The radiology department may have an acutely ill patient requiring priority.
- Procedures and/or tests that require completion prior to the radiologic exam:
  - A septic patient requires a series of tests to be performed within a designated timeframe (e.g., lactate level, blood cultures, antibiotics, and fluids).
  - Nausea or pain: Controlling patient nausea or pain prior to transport enhances patient comfort, improves patient cooperation, and increases radiology staff efficiency and patient safety.
- Oral contrast: The patient may not have consumed the required volume of contrast due to the patient experiencing nausea, vomiting, and/or pain.
- IV access: The nurse may face difficulty obtaining appropriate IV access suitable for IV contrast, or the saline lock the patient had is not patent.

- Test results: ED staff may be waiting for required lab results for the patient prior to leaving for a diagnostic exam (e.g., creatinine, glomerular filtration rate [GFR], urine pregnancy test, or beta-human chorionic gonadotropin [HCG]). Some exams will be canceled due to abnormal or unexpected lab results, while others may require additional patient intervention(s).

Fast Facts

Communication between ED and radiology staff is critical to quality patient care. Staff experience high levels of frustration when insufficient communication occurs. Taking time to communicate enhances work efficiency, decreases the wait time for results, and improves patient outcomes.

References

Joint Commission Center for Transforming Healthcare. (2013). *Improving transitions of care: Handoff communication*. Retrieved from https://www.qmo.amedd.army.mil/ptsafety/ArmyCTHPresentationApril2013pptx.pdf

The Joint Commission. (2017). *Sentinel alert event* (p. 58). Retrieved from https://www.jointcommission.org/en/resources/patient-safety-topics/sentinel-event/sentinel-event-alert-newsletters/sentinel-event-alert-58-inadequate-hand-off-communication/

World Health Organization. (2007). *Communication during patient handovers* (Vol. 1, p. 3). Retrieved from https://www.who.int/patientsafety/solutions/patientsafety/PS-Solution3.pdf?ua=1

32

Preparing ED Patients for Radiological Tests

Lynn Sayre Visser and Anna C. Montejano

Synchrony between the ED and radiology department ensures patient safety, efficient care, and the ability to meet core measure/time-sensitive treatment guidelines. Understanding what radiological diagnostic tests are commonly needed in the ED, and in how rapid of a manner, will help the radiology team to provide the highest level of care. A number of core measures/time-sensitive medical conditions require rapid patient intervention to save a life or minimize adverse outcomes.

In this chapter, you will discover:

1. How to identify four common radiological tests needed in the ED
2. How to recognize three core measure/time-sensitive medical conditions
3. Guidelines that should be met by radiology staff

COMMON ED RADIOLOGICAL PROCEDURES

The most common radiology procedures ordered in the ED that help determine the patient diagnosis include x-ray, computed tomography

(CT), ultrasound, magnetic resonance imaging (MRI), and nuclear medicine studies.

X-Ray

In some cases, an ED patient can go to radiology for films, but at other times a portable x-ray is necessary.

Common reasons for a portable x-ray include:

- Immediate verification of correct placement following endotracheal tube (ETT), central line insertion, and/or nasogastric tube placement.
- The patient is too unstable for transfer (e.g., cardiac dysrhythmias and/or hemodynamic instability).
- Postprocedural monitoring due to sedation (e.g., hip or shoulder relocation or fracture reduction and stabilization).
- Core measure/time-sensitive conditions requiring that multiple procedures/tests occur simultaneously (time is of the essence; the patient should not leave the ED).

Note: Prior to positioning a patient for a portable film, the patient's medical condition must be considered. For example, with a spinal cord injury, cervical spine immobilization must be maintained until medically cleared by a designated provider. Additionally, precautions must be taken to ensure hemodynamic stability.

Fast Facts

The ED provider requires quick radiological interpretation especially following intubation and/or central line placement to rule out a postprocedure complication and the need to provide vital treatment once placement is confirmed.

MRI

Common reasons for an MRI include:

- Evaluating for spinal cord compression or injury due to a herniated disc or tumor(s)
- A spinal infection caused by an abscess

Note: Even if the MRI patient screening is completed in the ED, the radiology staff will still verify for the possibility of internal/external metal objects (potential projectiles in the MRI), pain, claustrophobia, or contrast allergy and ensure any medical devices (e.g., ventilators, infusion pumps) are safe for the MRI scanner. MRI staff will also screen any ED staff who accompany the patient to the scanner for metal objects (e.g., keys, credit cards, hair barrettes, etc.).

CT

Common reasons for CT include:

- A neurological cause such as a change in level of consciousness to determine if the patient has a hemorrhagic versus ischemic stroke
- Diagnostics for a multitude of fractures, including those of the skull and facial bones

Note: Prioritize patients requiring CTs, so the sickest patients are treated first.

Ultrasound

Common reasons for ultrasound include:

- Rapid assessment for the possibility of a testicular torsion, ovarian torsion, or ectopic pregnancy requiring immediate surgical intervention as well as screening for deep vein thrombosis

Note: The patient with a rule-out ectopic pregnancy may require an indwelling catheter and/or IV fluids to fill the bladder prior to testing.

Nuclear Medicine

Common reasons for a nuclear medicine study include:

- Determination of a pulmonary embolus for patients with kidney impairment and/or hypersensitivity to contrast
- Diagnostics for a gastrointestinal bleed

Note: Following the study, recommendations for poststudy interventions should be relayed to the ED staff.

Fast Facts

Consider the need for pain management, control of anxiety, and/or sedation prior to radiology procedures. Advocate for the patient as needed.

BEFORE MOVING AN ED PATIENT

Many factors must be considered before determining if it is safe to move an ED patient. Some patients who are clinically fragile may need extra care, including:

- Intubated patients requiring continued patency of the airway and ventilator line management.
- Patients with a spinal cord injury.
- Restrained patients; loosening restraints causes concern that the patient may attempt to remove medical devices, intentionally or unintentionally (e.g., endotracheal tube, intravenous [IV] lines), or potentially harm self, staff, or others.
- Inotrope support such that repositioning would cause cardiovascular collapse.
- Patients with multiple lines and tubing (e.g., intravenous lines, central lines, drains, etc.).

Patient Safety Is First, Always

Following any radiological test or procedure, always think about patient safety.

- *Side rails:* Place the side rails up.
- *Gurney/bed height:* Leave the patient's gurney in a low position.
- *Equipment/lines:* Ensure when the patient is returned to the ED, communication with the ED staff takes place so interventions like cardiac monitoring, IV infusions, and so forth are restarted by the appropriate personnel and per facility policies.
- *Change in condition:* If the patient's status changes during the procedure, notify the ED nurse or physician immediately so that an intervention can be provided as necessary.
- *Postprocedure guidelines:* Upon return of an ED patient, any needed postprocedure positioning or follow-up care (e.g., fluid intake) should be conveyed to the ED staff.
- *Admission to floor:* If the patient is going to be admitted to the hospital floor directly following the radiology test, clear communication needs to take place between all involved to ensure system efficiency and patient comfort.

CORE MEASURES/TIME-SENSITIVE MEDICAL CONDITIONS

Acute myocardial infarction (AMI), stroke, sepsis, and pneumonia require timely intervention to reduce mortality and morbidity rates.

These cases require collaboration of multiple departments to meet patient needs. Most of these conditions are known as core measures, which are national initiatives used to determine the quality of hospital performance and patient care.

Acute Myocardial Infarction

Rapid identification of an AMI is critical to reduce mortality and morbidity rates. An immediate chest x-ray (CXR) rules out an aortic aneurysm since thrombolytic (e.g., tissue plasminogen activator, streptokinase, etc.) therapy is contraindicated in the presence of an aortic aneurysm. AMI treatment goals outlining the initial timeframe guidelines are shown in Table 32.1.

Table 32.1

Acute Myocardial Infarction Treatment Goals	
Timeframe	Treatment
Within 10 minutes of arrival	EKG
Upon arrival	Aspirin
Before giving a thrombolite	CXR
Within <30 minutes of arrival	Thrombolytic or cardiac catheterization lab
Within <90 minutes of arrival	Percutaneous coronary intervention (door-to-needle timeline)

CXR, chest x-ray
Source: Reproduced from Visser, L., & Montejano, A. (2019). *Fast facts for the triage nurse: An orientation and care guide* (2nd ed.). New York, NY: Springer Publishing Company.

Stroke

- A patient who exhibits signs and symptoms of a stroke requires a rapid head CT (to determine the type of stroke: hemorrhagic or ischemic) within timeframes established by the National Institutes of Neurological Disorders and Stroke (NINDS).
    - Knowing when the patient was *last seen normal* is critical in treatment decision-making for a patient to receive thrombolytic therapy.
    - Refer to Table 32.2: Treatment Timeframes for Stroke Care for guidelines.

- The head CT is time-sensitive so the medical provider can determine if the patient can receive fibrinolytic therapy (contraindicated for a hemorrhagic stroke).
  - Refer to Table 32.2 for guidelines.
  - Time zero for the purposes of radiology treatment begins as the patient enters the ED doors.
  - In some facilities, once an ischemic stroke is diagnosed, fibrinolytic therapy may even be started while the patient is in radiology.
  - Close communication between the ED, radiology, and pharmacy staff is critical for this to occur smoothly.

Table 32.2

Treatment Timeframes for Stroke Care

Timeframe	Treatment
Within 10 minutes of arrival	Perform a triage assessment Neurological screening ED medical provider evaluation
Within 15 minutes of arrival	Activate stroke team
Within 25 minutes of arrival	Obtain CT scan of head
Within 45 minutes of arrival	Head CT interpretation
Within 60 minutes of arrival	Determine candidacy for fibrinolytics Door-to-drug time
Within 3 hours of symptom onset	Begin post fibrinolytic pathway

Source: Reproduced from Visser, L., & Montejano, A. (2019). *Fast facts for the triage nurse: An orientation and care guide* (2nd ed.). New York, NY: Springer Publishing Company.

Sepsis

- Pneumonia, along with many other medical conditions, may lead to sepsis. The *initial screening* for sepsis takes place in the ED and requires two questions to be answered:
  1. Does the patient have an infection or suspicion of an infection?
  2. Is the patient taking antibiotics?
- If either of these questions results in a yes answer, the nurse continues in evaluating for systemic inflammatory response syndrome (SIRS) criteria, which involves consideration of the person's mental state, vital signs, white blood cell count, and blood glucose level.

- If the screening is positive (potential for sepsis), a radiological diagnostic test may lead to identifying the source of infection. For example, the CXR may indicate pneumonia, which will help the medical provider order appropriate antibiotics.
- An acutely ill septic patient may also require a stat portable CXR to confirm central line placement so that rapid fluid administration and antibiotics can be initiated as part of the sepsis treatment protocol.
- If the patient has changing vital signs while in radiology, notifying the ED staff of this change is critical. A patient may not meet SIRS criteria initially, but due to their change in presentation may become a candidate for sepsis treatment. Failure to treat a septic patient can lead to an adverse patient outcome.
- Pneumonia
  - A patient who arrives with symptoms of pneumonia needs a CXR as soon as possible so that the pneumonia core measure can be implemented.
  - Timely antibiotic administration is the essential component of this core measure with a goal of door-to-antibiotic time of fewer than 4 hours.
  - Prior to the administration of the antibiotic, two sets of blood cultures should be obtained.

Fast Facts

The importance of meeting the timelines with 100% efficiency not only provides evidence-based care but also demonstrates compliance with the requirements developed by The Joint Commission and the Center for Medicare and Medicaid Services.

Meeting timeframes for time-sensitive medical conditions requires intradepartmental teamwork, collaboration, and communication, which results in high-quality patient care.

Reference

Visser, L., & Montejano, A. (2019). *Fast facts for the triage nurse: An orientation and care guide* (2nd ed.). New York, NY: Springer Publishing Company.

Additional Resources

Albers, G. W., Marks, M. P., Kemp, S., Christensen, S., Tsai, J. P., Ortega-Gutierrez, S., & Lansberg, M. G. (2018). Thrombectomy for stroke at 6 to 16 hours with selection by perfusion imaging. *New England Journal of Medicine, 378*, 708–718. doi:10.1056/NEJMoa1713973

National Stroke Association. (n.d.). *Stroke resources.* Retrieved from http:// www.stroke.org/strokeresources?gclid=EAIaIQobChMIuPSrpYnX2wIV GNlkCh27MQ35EAAYASAAEgKm_vD_BwE

Nogueira, R. G., Jadhav, A. P., Haussen, D. C., Bonafe, A., Budzik, R. F., Bhuva, P., & Jovin, T. G. (2018). Thrombectomy 6 to 24 hours after stroke with a mismatch between deficit and infarct. *New England Journal of Medicine, 378*, 11–21. doi:10.1056/NEJMoa1706442

Visser, L., & Montejano, A. (2018). *Rapid access guide for triage and emergency nurses: Chief complaints with high risk presentations.* New York, NY: Springer Publishing Company.

33

Disaster Management

Valerie Aarne Grossman

Have you ever wondered what it would be like if you had to evacuate your hospital because of an approaching wildfire or mass flooding from a storm surge? Or what if you received hundreds of patients who needed imaging as a result of a mass casualty incident (MCI) like a bombing, mass shooting, or earthquake? Every radiology department should have an established disaster management plan that is practiced often and updated regularly.

In this chapter, you will discover:

1. Lessons learned from case studies of events around the world
2. Proper supply plans for disasters
3. The importance of planning and practicing drills

Throughout history, devastating events have occurred resulting in great suffering upon others.

Regulatory agencies, governmental agencies, and worldwide organizations have been vigilant in disaster management seeking best practice, educational opportunities, and interagency collaboration. The common goals include:

- Preparation (goals are to minimize the effect of a disaster by advanced education, supply warehousing, security evaluations, anticipate risks, etc.)

- Respond (identify the risk occurring, implement the established plan, safety/security, mobilize responding teams, continually reassessing needs of those affected, communication, etc.)
- Recover (may begin during the response phase and continue until the affected area is returned to a normal state of functioning)

Many agencies around the world are involved with disaster management. Some of them are:

- Centers for Disease Control and Prevention (CDC)
- Department of Homeland Security (DHS)
- Department of Health (DOH)
- Federal Emergency Management Agency (FEMA)
- National Academies of Science, Engineering, and Medicine (NASEM)
- National Incident Management System (NIMS)
- Nuclear Regulatory Commission (NRC)
- Occupational Safety and Health Administration (OSHA)
- Organisation for the Prohibition of Chemical Weapons (OPCW)
- Red Cross (American, International, etc.)
- The Joint Commission (TJC)
- World Health Organization (WHO)

Disasters can be categorized into similar events, including:

- Natural: Avalanches, droughts, wildfires, earthquakes, extreme heat/cold, hurricanes, tornadoes, storm surges, landslides/mudslides, volcano eruptions, floods, snowstorms, thunderstorms/lightning, tsunamis
- Society events: Active shooter, mass shooting incident, bomb explosion, biological attacks, chemical weapons, intentional or accidental contamination of food/water supply, hazardous material incidents, civil unrest, stampede, terror attack, pandemics, structure collapse, mass transit accidents, cybersecurity breach, loss of power, natural gas explosions, nuclear event, loss of communication capability (cell tower, satellite, etc.)

Some may think that disaster events only happen occasionally. In reality, these events have happened throughout world history. Some examples can be found in Table 33.1.

Table 33.1

Historical Disaster Events

Natural Disasters and Extreme Weather

- Hurricanes, tornadoes, blizzards, wildfires
- Flooding, storm surge, tsunami
- Earthquake, volcano eruption, mudslides
- **Historical Examples:**
  - 2005 Hurricane Katrina
  - 2010 Haiti earthquake
  - 2010 Mudslides in India
  - 2011 Christchurch (NZ) earthquake
  - 2011 Japan earthquake and tsunami
  - 2011 (62) tornadoes in a single day, central Alabama
  - 2012 Superstorm Sandy (both blizzard & hurricane)
  - 2017 Hurricanes Harvey, Irma, and Maria
  - 2018 Wildfire (California Camp Fire)
  - 2019 Hurricane Dorian

Violence

- Weapons of mass destruction
- Shooting incidents
- Bombs
- Vehicles used as weapons
- Civil unrest
- Cyberattacks
- **Historical Examples:**
  - 1788 NYC Doctors Mob Riot
    - 1st documented civil unrest w/ fatalities
  - 1840 University of Virginia
    - 1st documented school shooting
  - 1995 Oklahoma City Bombing
  - 1999 Columbine High School Massacre
  - 2001 9/11 terrorist attacks
  - 2004 Madrid train bombings
  - 2008 Taj Hotel terror attack, Mumbai
  - 2013 Boston Marathon Bombing
  - 2015 Paris, France: Suicide bombing and mass shooting
  - 2016 Nice, France: Truck driven into a crowd
  - 2019 Christchurch, NZ: Mosque terror attack
  - 2017 Buffalo, New York
    - Ransomware attack at Erie County Medical Center
  - 2017 Dallas, Texas
    - Cyberattack set off 156 emergency sirens
  - 2017 United Kingdom
    - Ransomware attack of 16 National Health Service hospitals

(continued)

Table 33.1

Historical Disaster Events (*continued*)

Accidental and Unintentional Disasters

- Nuclear events
- Explosions
- Mass transit accidents
- Structure collapse
- Human tragedy
- Stampede
- **Historical Examples:**
  - 1785 Hot air balloon crash Wimereux, France
    - 1st documented fatal aviation crash
  - 1986 Nuclear event Chernobyl, Soviet Ukraine
  - 1989 Hillsborough Stadium Collapse, England
  - 2012 Nuclear event, Fukushima, Japan
  - 2013 Factory collapse in Bangladesh
  - 2015 Pilgrimage stampede in Saudi Arabia

Chemical Weapons

- Chlorine
- Cyanide
- Hydrogen sulfide
- Mustard gas
- Nerve agents
- Sulfur mustard
- **Historical Examples:**
  - 1915 World War I in Belgium
    - 1st documented large-scale use of chlorine & mustard gas as a chemical weapon
  - 1995 Tokyo Subway (sarin gas)
  - 2011 Iraq & Syria (sarin, mustard gas, chlorine)
  - 2017 Australia (hydrogen sulfide attack)
  - 2018 Salisbury, England (nerve agent attack)

Biological Weapons

- Anthrax
- Bubonic plague
- Cholera
- Smallpox
- Salmonella *typhimurium*
- **Historical Examples:**
  - 1335 BC Middle East Hittite Plague
    - 1st documented biologic weapon
  - 1940 World War II Japan bombed China
    - Agents used included: bubonic plaque, cholera, smallpox, botulism, anthrax
  - 1984 Rajneeshee terror attack (food contamination Oregon)
  - 2001 U.S. mail (anthrax)

(*continued*)

Table 33.1

Historical Disaster Events (*continued*)

Pandemic

- Hemorrhagic fever
- Influenza
- Listeria
- Salmonellosis
- **Historical Examples:**
  - 1985 Listeria (food contamination) California
  - 2009 H1N1 pandemic
  - 2011 *E. coli* (food contamination) Germany
  - 2014 Ebola outbreak in West Africa
  - 2017 Listeria (food contamination) South Africa
  - 2019 COVID-19

Source: Data from Berger, F., Körner, M., Bernstein, M., Sodickson, A., Beenen, L., McLaughlin, P., & Bilow, R. (2016). Emergency imaging after a mass casualty incident: Role of the radiology department during training for and activation of a disaster management plan. *The British Journal of Radiology, 89*(1061), 20150984. doi:10.1259/bjr.20150984; Centers for Disease Control and Prevention. (2018a). *Past pandemics.* Retrieved from https://www.cdc.gov/cpr/readiness/hurricane_messages.htm; Centers for Disease Control and Prevention. (2018b). *Preparedness and safety messaging for hurricanes, flooding, and similar disasters.* Atlanta, GA: U.S. Department of Health and Human Services. Retrieved from https://www.cdc.gov/cpr/readiness/hurricane_messages.htm; Flammarion, C. (writing as Fulgence Marion). (1870). The necrology of aeronautics. In Cassell, Peter, & Galpin (Eds.), *Wonderful balloon ascents; or, the conquest of the skies* (pp. 181–186). Retrieved from https://en.wikisource.org/wiki/Wonderful_Balloon_Ascents/Part_2/Chapter_10; Goodwin Veenema, T. (2019). *Disaster nursing and emergency preparedness.* New York, NY: Springer Publishing Company; Grojec, W., & Coelho, C. (2018). *Chemical weapons: A deadly history. Radio Free Europe.* Retrieved from https://www.rferl.org/a/history-of-chemical-weapons/29184063.html; Haygood, T. (2018). Including radiology in emergency plans is critical. *RSNA News, 28*(8), 10–12. Retrieved from https://www.rsna.org/uploadedFiles/RSNA/Content/News/2018/08_August/August2018.pdf; Organisation for the Prohibition of Chemical Weapons. (n.d.). *History looking back helps us look forward.* Retrieved from https://www.opcw.org/about-us/history; Richmond Enquirer. (1840). *Painful Occurrence, 37*(58), 2. Retrieved from https://chroniclingamerica.loc.gov/lccn/sn84024735/1840-11-17/ed-1/seq-2/#words=Painful+Occurrence; Schoeberl, R. (2018). CBRNE weapons & Islamic state—A bad combination. *DomPrep Journal, 14*(4), 6–8; Sen, D. (2013). Coping in a calamity: Radiology during the cloudburst at Leh. *Indian Journal of Radiology Imaging, 23*(1), 106–109. Retrieved from http://www.ijri.org/text.asp?2013/23/1/106/113629; Snair, J. (2018). Improving local health department cybersecurity. *DomPrep Journal, 14*(4), 9–15; Sutherland, S. (2019, February). 135 minutes. *National Fire Protection Association Journal.* Retrieved from https://www.nfpa.org/News-and-Research/Publications-and-media/NFPA-Journal/2019/January-February-2019/POV/Perspectives; Török, T. J., Tauxe, R. V., Wise, R. P., Livengood, J. R., Sokolow, R., Mauvais, S., & Foster, L. R. (1997). A large community outbreak of salmonellosis caused by Intentional Contamination of Restaurant Salad Bars. *JAMA, 278*(5), 389–395. doi:10.1001/jama.1997.03550050051033; Trevisanato, S. (2007). The 'Hittite plague', an epidemic of tularemia and the first record of biological warfare. *Medical Hypothesis, 69*(6), 1163–1388. doi:10.1016/j.mehy.2007.03.012

Regardless of the disaster, many response actions and goals will be similar. Hospitals may have established disaster management plans; however, radiology departments are often left out of those plans. It is essential for all radiology departments to have their own specific disaster plan for the "what ifs" that can occur. These plans should be updated regularly and practiced often (including drills during the night, weekends, etc.). Case studies exist from organizations that have experienced disaster events. Reviewing these events can help each radiology department to consider details as they may pertain to their own environments.

2010 Mudslide in Leh, India, Following a Heavy Downpour

- The region averages 4 inches of rainfall per year. A cloudburst occurred at *midnight*, and showered the region with 14 inches of rain within 2 hours, creating flash floods, mudflows, and debris rivers.
- Victims, unaware of this disaster, were unable to avoid the path of destruction.
  - Many survivors were partially buried in mud or under debris.
- The Sonam Nurboo Memorial Hospital was closest to the mudslide and became inoperable due to sludge and flooding.
- The Army Hospital of Leh (210 beds) was the next closest hospital and received 549 patients.
- Seventy-one towns were damaged; 9,000 people were impacted.
- Impact on radiology:
  - In the first 48 hours post event, the radiology department imaged a volume of patients normally seen in a 5-day period.
  - Due to patient conditions (unconscious, children separated from adults, etc.), patient identification, documentation, and communication were difficult.
    - Identifying numbers were written on the patient's forehead or wrist and were used to identify radiological studies and medical records.
  - Prompt imaging and triage of presenting patients allowed for expedited and accurate patient assessment, organized delivery of patient care, and accurate disposition (surgery, discharge, etc.).
    - A radiologist worked alongside ED triage and prioritized the imaging studies needed (plain films, focused assessment with sonography in trauma [FAST], CT, etc.).
    - The reading radiologist went directly to the ordering care provider to deliver the image interpretation to avoid errors in communication from occurring.
  - Patients were difficult to identify, and hallways were used for patients on stretchers, making it more difficult for radiology staff to find and identify patients who had imaging ordered.

- Many patients sustained eye injuries from the mudslide and had at least temporary blindness, making their conditions more complicated.
- Patients were often caked with mud, making wound assessment and anatomical identification difficult. Imaging studies were initially slowed down, as the mud-caked clothing made equipment dirty and required more cleaning between patients (patients were soon undressed and cleaned prior to going for imaging studies, thus keeping equipment cleaner).
- A portable ultrasound machine was stationed in the ICU to reduce the time wasted in transporting patients to/from ICU to radiology.
- Unidirectional patient flow was initiated in radiology so that all patients entered the department from one end and exited the radiology department from the other end (Gupta, Khanna, & Majumdar, 2012; Sen, 2013; Singh & Bhatnagar, 2016).

Fast Facts

Patients should be properly identified and prepared for their imaging studies so patient throughput can be expedited, avoiding delay of care for the high volume of patients waiting to be treated.

2011 Christchurch, New Zealand, Earthquake

- Christchurch Public Hospital (CPH) and Christchurch Women's Hospital (CWH) occupy the same physical site but are separate buildings.
- The CWH ground floor radiology department consisted of one x-ray room, four ultrasound rooms, a radiologist reading suite, and a fetal medicine scanning and consulting room.
- The CPH's first-level radiology department consisted of three CT scanners, two DSA rooms, one MRI, five ultrasound rooms, and general x-ray rooms.
- Without warning, a 6.3 magnitude earthquake occurred on February 22, 2011, at 12:51 p.m. and lasted 37 seconds. There were 10 aftershocks in the next 14 hours, up to magnitudes of 5.9.
- In the first 24 hours, 182 people died, and 6,500 people were injured in the community.
- The hospitals activated both their internal and external disaster plans.

- CWH was built with "state-of-the-art" seismic upgrades in 2005; however, geotechnical failures occurred, including widespread damage to the hospital structure:
  - Cracks in the ceilings, floors, walls, and stairwells
  - Flooding of the tunnels
  - Damage to the roof, boiler stack, medical equipment, and elevators
  - Loss of electrical power and telephone communication
- The earthquake resulted in the evacuation of 350 patients from Christchurch Hospital (600+ bed facility) in 35 minutes, while their ED remained open.
- Radiology department was impacted by:
  - Loss of power (power outages as well as the loss of the backup generator)
  - Interrupted communication capabilities and flooding of the department
  - Malfunction of the sprinkler system caused flooding of the scanning room and ultrasound room
  - During the first 5 to 12 hours after the earthquake, only portable x-rays and ultrasound imaging were available to the ED
  - Ultrasound units were found to be too large and did not perform well with the interruption in their power source, so radiologists relied on the FAST scans
  - No images from those initial hours were saved; however, a verbal report was given directly to the ED physician and a brief handwritten radiologist report created
  - Nuclear medicine received no damage; CT scanners were operable after initial 12 hours (de Ryke, 2012; Gregan, Balasingam, & Butler, 2016; Mitrani-Reiser et al., 2011)

2011 EF-5 Tornado Directly Hit St. Johns-Mercy Hospital (367 Beds) in Joplin, Missouri

- Tornado's path was 14 miles by 1 mile in size, winds exceeded 200 mph, 8,000 buildings were destroyed in the community, 18,000 vehicles were destroyed, 1,000 people were injured, and 161 people were killed.
- St. Johns-Mercy Hospital (367 licensed beds) received a 24-minute advanced warning: The tornado hovered over the hospital for 45 seconds. They were in the process of implementing their EMR and purposely kept census down.
- Around 183 hospitalized patients were evacuated within 90 minutes of the event. Items used to transport patients out of the hospital included backboards, chairs, wheelchairs, doors, sheets, mattresses, and evacuation sleds.
- Hospital structures were severely affected:
  - Windows exploded.

- Roof, walls, and floors torn or blown away.
- The building shifted 4 inches off of its foundation.
- Generator failed, and communication capabilities were lost (computers, telephones, Internet, pagers, overhead announcing system, etc.).
- Water/gas/sewer lines broke.
- Equipment was destroyed (helicopter, disaster trailer, heating, ventilation, and air conditioning [HVAC], vehicles, etc.).

- A 4-day cache of supplies was depleted within 4 hours of the disaster event.
- Water was flooding the hospital floors (3- to 6-inch deep), natural gas was filling the air, and raw sewage flowed through the facility.
- Within a few hours, 135 doctors arrived at St. Johns-Mercy to help patients as well as countless other employees.
- During recovery and rebuilding, employees continued to receive their regular paychecks.
- Effects on radiology:
  - Portable x-ray machines became airborne.
  - The wind propelled debris and people; humans were unable to remain in safe hiding places.
  - Fire axes were used to obtain medications from the locked electronic medication cabinets.
  - X-ray films were found up to 100 miles away (Adler & Bauer, 2016; Reynolds, 2011).

2013 Boston Marathon Bombing

- Perpetrators exploded two homemade bombs at the finish line of the race, injuring 275+ people.
- About 90 of the injured people were treated at three hospitals.
- Hospitals initiated disaster plans, and staff were mobilized into work.
- Demands on radiology departments:
  - 50% of patients required chest x-rays.
  - 25% of patients required CT scans.
  - 23% of patients required pelvic x-rays.
  - 18% of patients required focused abdominal ultrasound in trauma (FAST; Gates et al., 2014).

Fast Facts

It is common during a disaster for organizations to run short on supplies such as pens, paper, cleaning supplies, linen, personal protective equipment (PPE), food, water, flashlights, and batteries.

263 Chapter 33 Disaster Management

2017 Cyberattack Upon the Erie County Medical Center (ECMC) in Buffalo, NY

- Cyberattacks on healthcare organizations have skyrocketed since the implementation of the "meaningful use" requirements of the 2009 Health Information Technology for Economic and Clinical Health (HITECH) Act
- Federal Bureau of Investigation (FBI): 4,000 ransomware attacks worldwide between January 1, 2016, and May 17, 2020.
- ECMC practiced downtime drills as part of their disaster management plan, which included "computer-less" operation drills (prior to this attack).
- At 2 a.m. on April 9, 2017, computer screens at ECMC flashed with a message that read: "*What happened to your files?*" The hackers demanded a ransom in bitcoins—equivalent to $44,000—to unlock them.
- *SamSam*, the attacking force, exploits system vulnerabilities (administrative passwords) and can evade antivirus protection.
- About 6,000 computers were locked down, affecting the 600-plus-bed hospital and 390-bed nursing home.
  - ECMC went 13 days without computers, was disconnected from the Internet for 45 days, and reverted to paper charting for 6 weeks during their recovery.
- Impact on radiology:
  - Paper requisitions were used to order imaging studies.
  - Initially, radiologists viewed images directly on the machines but ran out of local storage after a few days.
    - Images were then printed on film, and radiologists used lightboxes to read studies and handwrote reports.
  - At least one radiologist remained on duty 24-7 to read scans directly from the CT scanner.
  - Clerical staff hand-delivered radiology reports to the ordering provider.
  - Additional staff were scheduled to assist with additional workflow created by lack of computers.
  - Extra efforts were put into place to maintain staff morale during this difficult 6-week period.
  - During the 6-week recovery, laptop computers with wireless hot spots were supplied to key departments (ED, ICU, radiology, etc.).
  - Financial services were impacted, billers' and coders' workflow was severely slowed, and collections were taking up to 45 days.

- Historical images obtained prior to the attack were archived on the Western New York Clinical Information Exchange (HealtheLink; Advisory Board, 2017; Defino, 2018; Millard, 2017; Pugh & Dameff, 2017; Slabodkin, 2017).

Fast Facts

During mock disaster drills, it is important for staff to drill without power, water, computers, telephones, and other "modern" conveniences. Drills should happen regularly and prepare staff for the "worst-case scenario."

2017 Las Vegas Mass Shooting

- Perpetrator fired 1,000+ rounds in less than 15 minutes into a crowd of 22,000 people.
- Most of the 851 injured patients were treated at three hospitals.
    - About 422 of those patients had gunshot wounds (GSWs), and most required a CT scan.
- Hospitals ran out of supplies, including chest tubes, IV solution, ventilators, and cleaning supplies.
- Bottlenecks and their workarounds:
    - Waiting for Pyxis to identify a person's fingerprint slowed down patient care (a pharmacist removed supplies of medications and dispensed them).
    - Transporting to/from CT scan (CT tech remained at control desk, nurses transported monitored patients to CT/moved patient on and off table).
    - Transporting patients to/from x-ray department and radiologist interpretation (radiologist, radiologic technologist, and portable x-ray machine when to ED and performed bedside imaging and interpretation) (Lozada et al., 2019; Menes, Tintinalli, & Plaster, 2017).

Lessons can be learned from reviewing case studies, reading articles, or attending live presentations by those who have experienced firsthand a disaster. Each person should consider how they would be able to respond, should such a disaster occur at their own institution. Refer to Table 33.2 for a list of generalized lessons learned by others.

Table 33.2

Generalized Lessons Learned From Past Disaster Events	
Leadership	■ Must be present on the front line, stay calm and optimistic, and be informative ■ Frequent updates for staff will keep staff organized, reduce inaccurate rumors, and keep fears at a minimum ■ Leadership will be the role model for staff; staff must be able to portray calm, safety, and organized response to the patients ■ Leadership must understand the emotional response of staff and be ready to assist ■ Manage the media coverage and what is reported
Safety/security	■ Maintain crowd control ■ Keep supplies in a secure location (to avoid looting) ■ Surround damaged buildings with tall fences (6 inches tall) ■ Have portable illuminated signs to identify exits ■ Establish a security rapid response team that will maintain all security details during and after a disaster ■ Armed security may be needed ■ ID badges are often lost during a disaster: Staff should also have wallet-size ID cards ■ Security cameras should be on backup power ■ Control parking lot and influx of patients and visitors
Disaster plan	■ Must include radiology department ■ Must be updated regularly and practiced often ■ Must practice on all shifts (24-7/365) ■ All levels of staff must participate in disaster planning including senior leadership, physicians, and all front-line staff
Electrical	■ Protect generators from flooding ■ All areas of radiology must be on backup generator ■ Ample supply of flashlights, headlamps, and batteries ■ Established plan in case of generator failure ■ Heliport lights should be on backup power
Communication	■ Up-to-date phone lists (departments, employees, vendors, etc.) ■ Available portable phones (satellite, Wi-Fi, wireless radios, etc.) ■ When calling for help, be clear with location and the issue in need ■ Radiology a command center, with one central phone number ■ Provide solar charging stations for cell phone and radio batteries

(continued)

Table 33.2

Generalized Lessons Learned From Past Disaster Events (*continued*)

Medical records	■ Must have backup paper process in place in case computers go down ■ PACS systems may become unavailable
Patient identification	■ If ID bands not available, use permanent marker on patient's skin
Patient preparation	■ Remove clothing (especially if wet or muddy) ■ Obtain history prior to entering imaging room
Evacuation plan	■ Should be practiced often ■ Predetermined muster stations ■ Backup plans (i.e., EMS not available, equipment not available, etc.) ■ Designate one stairway for "up" and one for "down" traffic ■ Hard copy of policies and procedures
Supplies	■ Average PAR is 2 to 5 days: During a disaster, most run out of supplies in 4 to 48 hours. ■ Many report running out of pens, paper, water, food, flashlights, batteries, cleaning supplies, first aid supplies, linen, PPE (goggles, gowns, masks, gloves), orthopedic supplies (splints, crutches, casting material, etc.) ■ Radiology should have emergency kits that include flashlights, batteries, handheld radios ■ Oxygen lines and portable oxygen tanks may become in short supply ■ Identification vests for staff ■ Drug-dispensing machines are locked and unable to be opened (have keys available for supervisors, use sledgehammer to open, or have pharmacist present with supply of medications)
Staffing	■ Double radiologist on duty (in case staff are not permitted to leave, one team can sleep while the other team works) ■ Staff technologist and nursing staff at 150% of normal ■ Radiologists may be able to read studies remotely ■ Some radiologists/technologists may relocate to the ED bedside to facilitate imaging and interpretation ■ Provide debriefing after events for staff, have EAP available ■ Connect with staff quickly, provide for their wellbeing ■ Have a plan for responding volunteers ■ Have a team ready to provide emotional support (chaplains, social workers, EAP, etc.)

Table 33.2

Generalized Lessons Learned From Past Disaster Events
(continued)

Patient flow	■ Establish unidirectional patient flow through the radiology department: One door for incoming patients and a different door for outgoing patients ■ Assign staff to streamline patient flow (i.e., one technologist obtains image, another person transports patients, another cleans equipment, IV placement, etc.)
Equipment protection	■ Imaging equipment is easily damaged by temperature variation (hot/cold), moisture, dust, flooding, vibrations (earthquake) ■ If main radiology department has damaged equipment, consider equipment in other departments (clinic x-ray machines, operating room c-arms, etc.) ■ MRI suites are closed until risk of quench has passed ■ Prioritize patients needing imaging, life-threatening situations first
Approaching storm	■ Dictate all studies as soon as possible ■ Stock all rooms with plenty of supplies ■ Review disaster plan with all staff ■ Relocate portable equipment on upper floors in case of elevator loss ■ Protect imaging equipment from water damage, flooding, power outage
Patient evacuation	■ Remove IV tubing and bags if possible ■ Have fathers carry newborn babies ■ Have patients put on their shoes, take warm coats, dress appropriately ■ Designate one staircase for "up" traffic and one for "down" traffic ■ Log where patients are sent ■ EMS may not always be available to assist during an evacuation: Private cars, trucks, or school/public buses may be utilized

EAP, employee assistance program; EMS, emergency medical service; PACS, picture archiving and communication system; PPE, personal protective equipment.
Source: Adler, E., & Bauer, L. (2016, May 11). Joplin tornado of 2011: In St. John's medical center, heroism in the face of horror. *The Kansas City Star*. Retrieved from https://www.kansascity.com/news/local/article64775907.html; Advisory Board. (2017, May 25). *Today's daily briefing: At 2 a.m. on a Sunday, a hospital was hacked. Here's how it kept key departments operating.* Retrieved from https://www.advisory.com/daily-briefing/2017/05/25/ecmc-hack; Defino, T. (2018). Prepare for ransomware attack with archived forms, offline records, and constant practice. *Report on Patient Privacy, 18*(4). Retrieved from https://assets.hcca-info.org/Portals/0/PDFs/Resources/

Fast Facts

Ask yourself how would your radiology department react if any of these disasters happened to you.
Are you ready for these events? What more can you do now to prepare?

Rpt_Privacy/2018/RPP0418.pdf?ver=2018-04-04-104924-570; Department of Homeland Security. (2018a). *Disasters and emergencies.* Retrieved from https://www .ready.gov/be-informed; Department of Homeland Security. (2018b). *Emergency response plan.* Retrieved from https://www.ready.gov/business/implementation/ Emergency; Department of Homeland Security. (2019). *FEMA national response framework* (4th ed.). Retrieved from https://www.fema.gov/media-library/assets/ documents/117791; de Ryke, R. (2012). The Christchurch earthquake: Ultrasound in a mass trauma event. *Australasian Journal of Ultrasound in Medicine, 15*(3), 78–81. doi:10.1002/j.2205-0140.2012.tb00010.x ; Gates, J. D., Arabian, S., Biddinger, P., Blansfield, J., Burke, P., Chung, S., &Yaffe, M. B. (2014). The initial response to the Boston marathon bombing: Lessons learned to prepare for the next disaster. *Annals of Surgery, 260*(6), 960–966. doi:10.1097/SLA.0000000000000914; Gregan, J., Balasingam, A., & Butler, A. (2016). Radiology in the Christchurch earthquake of 22 February 2011: Challenges, interim processes and clinical priorities. *Journal of Medical Imaging and Radiation Oncology, 60*(2), 172–181. doi:10.1111/1754-9485.12315; Gupta, P., Khanna, A., & Majumdar, S. (2012). Disaster management in flash floods in leh (ladakh): A case study. *Indian Journal of Community Medicine, 37*(3), 185–190. doi:10.4103/0970-0218.99928; Lozada, M., Cai, S., Li, M., Davidson, S., Nix, J., & Ramsey, G. (2019). The Las Vegas mass shooting: An analysis of blood component administration and blood bank donations. *Journal of Trauma and Acute Care Surgery, 86*(1), 128–133. doi:10.1097/ TA.0000000000002089; Menes, K., Tintinalli, J., & Plaster, L. (2017, November 3). How one Las Vegas ED saved hundreds of lives after the worst mass shooting in U.S. History. *Emergency Physicians Monthly.* Retrieved from https://epmonthly.com/article/ not-heroes-wear-capes-one-las-vegas-ed-saved-hundreds-lives-worst-mass-shooting-u-s-history/; Millard, W. (2017). Where bits and bytes meet flesh and blood. *Annals of Emergency Medicine, 70*(3), A17–A21. doi:10.1016/j.annemergmed.2017.07.008; Mitrani-Reiser, J., Kirsch, T., Jacques, C., Giovinazzi, S., McIntosh, J., & Wilson, T. (2011). Response of the regional health care system to the 22nd February 2011, Christchurch Earthquake, NZ. *World Conferences on Earthquake Engineering.* Retrieved from https://www.iitk.ac.in/nicee/wcee/article/WCEE2012_4569.pdf; Pugh, J., & Dameff, C. (2017, October 17). What to do when cyber attack strikes the emergency department. *Acepnow.com.* Retrieved from https://www.acepnow.com/article/cyber-attack-strikes-emergency-department/2/?singlepage=1; Reynolds, M. (2011). *The Joplin Tornado: The hospital story and lessons learned.* Retrieved from https://cdn.ymaws.com/ www.leadingagemissouri.org/resource/resmgr/annual_conference/wednesday_joplin _tornado_les.pdf; Sen, D. (2013). Coping in a calamity: Radiology during the cloudburst at Leh. *Indian Journal of Radiology Imaging, 23*(1), 106–109. Retrieved from http://www .ijri.org/text.asp?2013/23/1/106/113629; Singh, G. K., & Bhatnagar, A. (2016). Cloud burst in Leh: Pattern of casualties; challenges faced and recommendations based on the management of such natural disaster at multi-specialty hospital. *International Journal of Health System and Disaster Management, 4,* 97–101

References

Adler, E., & Bauer, L. (2016, May 11). Joplin tornado of 2011: In St. John's medical center, heroism in the face of horror. *The Kansas City Star*. Retrieved from https://www.kansascity.com/news/local/article64775907.html

Advisory Board. (2017, May 25). *Today's daily briefing: At 2 a.m. on a Sunday, a hospital was hacked. Here's how it kept key departments operating.* Retrieved from https://www.advisory.com/daily-briefing/2017/05/25/ecmc-hack

Berger, F., Körner, M., Bernstein, M., Sodickson, A., Beenen, L., McLaughlin, P., & Bilow, R. (2016). Emergency imaging after a mass casualty incident: Role of the radiology department during training for and activation of a disaster management plan. *The British Journal of Radiology, 89*(1061), 20150984. doi:10.1259/bjr.20150984

Centers for Disease Control and Prevention. (2018a). *Past pandemics.* Retrieved from https://www.cdc.gov/flu/pandemic-resources/basics/past-pandemics.html

Centers for Disease Control and Prevention. (2018b). *Preparedness and safety messaging for hurricanes, flooding, and similar disasters.* Atlanta, GA: U.S. Department of Health and Human Services. Retrieved from https://www.cdc.gov/cpr/readiness/hurricane_messages.htm

Defino, T. (2018). Prepare for ransomware attack with archived forms, offline records, and constant practice. *Report on Patient Privacy, 18*(4). Retrieved from https://assets.hcca-info.org/Portals/0/PDFs/Resources/Rpt_Privacy/2018/RPP0418.pdf?ver=2018-04-04-104924-570

Department of Homeland Security. (2018a). *Disasters and emergencies.* Retrieved from https://www.ready.gov/be-informed

Department of Homeland Security. (2018b). *Emergency response plan.* Retrieved from https://www.ready.gov/business/implementation/emergency

Department of Homeland Security. (2019). *FEMA national response framework* (4th ed.). Retrieved from https://www.fema.gov/media-library/assets/documents/117791

de Ryke, R. (2012). The Christchurch earthquake: Ultrasound in a mass trauma event. *Australasian Journal of Ultrasound in Medicine, 15*(3), 78–81. doi:10.1002/j.2205-0140.2012.tb00010.x

Flammarion, C. (writing as Fulgence Marion). (1870). The necrology of aeronautics. In Cassell, Peter, & Galpin (Eds.), *Wonderful balloon ascents; or, the conquest of the skies* (pp. 181–186). Retrieved from https://en.wikisource.org/wiki/Wonderful_Balloon_Ascents/Part_2/Chapter_10

Gates, J. D., Arabian, S., Biddinger, P., Blansfield, J., Burke, P., Chung, S., & Yaffe, M. B. (2014). The initial response to the Boston marathon bombing: Lessons learned to prepare for the next disaster. *Annals of Surgery, 260*(6), 960–966. doi:10.1097/SLA.0000000000000914

Goodwin Veenema, T. (2019). *Disaster nursing and emergency preparedness.* New York, NY: Springer Publishing Company.

Gregan, J., Balasingam, A., & Butler, A. (2016). Radiology in the Christchurch earthquake of 22 February 2011: Challenges, interim processes and clinical priorities. *Journal of Medical Imaging and Radiation Oncology, 60*(2), 172–181. doi:10.1111/1754-9485.12315

Grojec, W., & Coelho, C. (2018). Chemical weapons: A deadly history. *Radio Free Europe*. Retrieved from https://www.rferl.org/a/history-of-chemical-weapons/29184063.html

Gupta, P., Khanna, A., & Majumdar, S. (2012). Disaster management in flash floods in leh (ladakh): A case study. *Indian Journal of Community Medicine, 37*(3), 185–190. doi:10.4103/0970-0218.99928

Haygood, T. (2018). Including radiology in emergency plans is critical. *RSNA News, 28*(8), 10–12. Retrieved from https://www.rsna.org/uploadedFiles/RSNA/Content/News/2018/08_August/August2018.pdf

Lozada, M., Cai, S., Li, M., Davidson, S., Nix, J., & Ramsey, G. (2019). The Las Vegas mass shooting: An analysis of blood component administration and blood bank donations. *Journal of Trauma and Acute Care Surgery, 86*(1), 128–133. doi:10.1097/TA.0000000000002089

Menes, K., Tintinalli, J., & Plaster, L. (2017, November 3). How one Las Vegas ED saved hundreds of lives after the worst mass shooting in U.S. History. *Emergency Physicians Monthly*. Retrieved from https://epmonthly.com/article/not-heroes-wear-capes-one-las-vegas-ed-saved-hundreds-lives-worst-mass-shooting-u-s-history/

Millard, W. (2017). Where bits and bytes meet flesh and blood. *Annals of Emergency Medicine, 70*(3), A17–A21. doi:10.1016/j.annemergmed.2017.07.008

Mitrani-Reiser, J., Kirsch, T., Jacques, C., Giovinazzi, S., McIntosh, J., & Wilson, T. (2011). Response of the regional health care system to the 22nd February 2011, Christchurch Earthquake, NZ. *World Conferences on Earthquake Engineering*. Retrieved from https://www.iitk.ac.in/nicee/wcee/article/WCEE2012_4569.pdf

Organisation for the Prohibition of Chemical Weapons. (n.d.). *History looking back helps us look forward*. Retrieved from https://www.opcw.org/about-us/history

Pugh, J., & Dameff, C. (2017, October 17). What to do when cyber attack strikes the emergency department. *Acepnow.com*. Retrieved from https://www.acepnow.com/article/cyber-attack-strikes-emergency-department/2/?singlepage=1

Reynolds, M. (2011). *The Joplin Tornado: The hospital story and lessons learned*. Retrieved from https://cdn.ymaws.com/www.leadingagemissouri.org/resource/resmgr/annual_conference/wednesday_joplin_tornado_les.pdf

Richmond Enquirer. (1840). *Painful Occurrence, 37*(58), 2. Retrieved from https://chroniclingamerica.loc.gov/lccn/sn84024735/1840-11-17/ed-1/seq-2/#words=Painful+Occurrence

Schoeberl, R. (2018). CBRNE weapons & Islamic state—A bad combination. *DomPrep Journal, 14*(4), 6–8.

Sen, D. (2013). Coping in a calamity: Radiology during the cloudburst at Leh. *Indian Journal of Radiology Imaging, 23*(1), 106–109. Retrieved from http://www.ijri.org/text.asp?2013/23/1/106/113629

Singh, G. K., & Bhatnagar, A. (2016). Cloud burst in Leh: Pattern of casualties; challenges faced and recommendations based on the management of such natural disaster at multi-specialty hospital. *International Journal of Health System and Disaster Management, 4*, 97–101.

Slabodkin, G. (2017, May 15). Cyber-attack on Erie County Medical Center was ransomware. *HealthData Management*. Retrieved from https://www.healthdatamanagement.com/news/ransomware-caused-cyber-attack-at-erie-county-medical-center

Snair, J. (2018). Improving local health department cybersecurity. *DomPrep Journal, 14*(4), 9–15.

Sutherland, S. (2019, February). 135 minutes. *National Fire Protection Association Journal*. Retrieved from https://www.nfpa.org/News-and-Research/Publications-and-media/NFPA-Journal/2019/January-February-2019/POV/Perspectives

Török, T. J., Tauxe, R. V., Wise, R. P., Livengood, J. R., Sokolow, R., Mauvais, S., . . . Foster, L. R. (1997). A large community outbreak of salmonellosis caused by Intentional Contamination of Restaurant Salad Bars. *JAMA, 278*(5), 389–395. doi:10.1001/jama.1997.03550050051033

Trevisanato, S. (2007). The 'Hittite plague', an epidemic of tularemia and the first record of biological warfare. *Medical Hypothesis, 69*(6), 1163–1388. doi:10.1016/j.mehy.2007.03.012

VII

Emerging Areas of
Radiology Nursing

34

Orientation, Point-of-Care Testing, Certification

Valerie Aarne Grossman

Radiology nursing will require the nurse to learn new skills, practice a wide variety of competencies, and continually grow professionally. Radiology departments often have a smaller compliment of nurses, so individual growth, professionalism, and teamwork development are essential.

In this chapter, you will discover:

1. Proper job orientation
2. Point-of-care testing for the radiology nurse
3. Certification in radiology nursing

Creating a high-functioning team of nurses begins with hiring the best candidates available for the right available positions. Each organization may have a different process for recruiting top talent; all should have the same goal of finding the best candidates. Recruiting new staff and retention of current quality employees should receive the highest level of attention from leadership.

For a complete resource on radiology nursing recruiting, orientation, and retention, refer to *Advanced Practice and Leadership in Radiology Nursing* by Kathleen A. Gross (2020), published by Springer Nature.

NURSING ORIENTATION

The orientation for each new nurse to the radiology environment will be developed based on the services provided and the patient population of the organization. Because the role of a radiology nurse is independent, many departments will recruit nurses with solid experience in critical care. Radiology nurses must have an expert command of patient care under difficult circumstances (patient acuity, fast-paced, different sets of information to synthesize, all age groups, etc.). To have a successful orientation program, each department should have:

- Strong leadership with clear team goals (Grossman, 2013)
- Skilled preceptors with sincere passion for mentoring
- Well-defined orientation objectives for each modality the nurse may be called to
- Ample time for each modality
  - May need 160 to 320 hours of orientation for IR procedures
  - May need 40 hours of orientation for individual modalities (i.e., CT, MRI, etc.)
- Checklists and competency documentation of stated orientation objectives
- Registration in hospital-offered classes (i.e., advanced cardiac life support [ACLS], telemetry, critical care, etc.)
- Weekly meetings with manager, preceptor, and orientee to discuss successes and hurdles of orientation progression
- Postorientation evaluation (Sousa, 2013)

POINT-OF-CARE TESTING

Bedside testing has changed over the past decade, and, in many states, it may be heavily regulated. The radiology nurse may need to be proficient in the following point-of-care testing techniques:

- Blood glucose
- Urine pregnancy
- Serum creatinine, blood urea nitrogen (BUN), estimated glomerular filtration rate (eGFR)—for contrast decisions
- Handheld Doppler for checking pulses, intravenous (IV) placement, and the like
- Activated clotting time (for interventional radiology procedural care)

The nurse will be required to follow the guidelines as established by governing agencies and organizational policy.

CERTIFICATION IN RADIOLOGY NURSING

A goal for all radiology nurses should be membership in a national nursing organization such as the Association for Radiologic & Imaging Nursing. If a radiology department specializes in a type of patient care (neurointerventional, vascular, oncology, pediatric, cardiology, etc.), the nurse should consider belonging to more than one nursing organization. This will allow the nurse access to the most up-to-date information as well as networking with other nurses who have a similar practice. As each nurse grows in their own practice, achieving certification is essential. To be eligible to take the certification exam in radiology nursing, one must:

- Possess a current, active registered nurse license in good standing in their state or the international licensure equivalent
- Have practiced in the radiology setting for a minimum of 2,000 hours in the previous 3 years
- Obtained 30 contact hours of approved continuing education within the previous 24 months, with a minimum of 15 hours specifically related to radiology nursing

Once obtained, certification is valid for 4 years from the date of passing the exam.

Fast Facts

The Radiologic Nursing Certification Board offers the certification exam for radiology nursing. More information can be found at https://www.certifiedradiologynurse.org.

References

Gross, K. A. (2020). *Advanced practice and leadership in radiology nursing.* Retrieved from https://www.springer.com/gp/book/9783030326784

Grossman, V. A. (2013). Teamwork essentials: Success in the radiology environment. *Journal of Radiology Nursing, 32*(3), 139–140. doi:10.1016/j.jradnu.2013.03.002

Sousa, M. (2013). Management and leadership: An agile approach to new nurse orientation: How one hospital created a sustainable orientation plan for newly hired radiology nurses. *Journal of Radiology Nursing, 32*(1), 45–47.

Abbreviations

ACLS	Advanced cardiac life support
ACR	American College of Radiology (www.acr.org)
ACT	Activated clotting time
ACTH	Adrenocorticotropic hormone
ADH	Atypical ductal hyperplasia
AIH	Alcohol-induced hypoglycemia
ALARA	As low as reasonably achievable
AMI	Acute myocardial infarction
Anti-Xa	Anti-factor Xa assay
AORN	Association of periOperative Registered Nurses (www.aorn.org)
aPTT	Activated partial thromboplastin time
ARIN	Association for Radiologic & Imaging Nursing (www.arinursing.org)
ARRA	American Recovery and Reinvestment Act of 2009 (https://www.govinfo.gov/content/pkg/BILLS-111hr1enr/pdf/BILLS-111hr1enr.pdf)
ASA	American Society of Anesthesiologists
AVF	Arteriovenous fistula
AVJ	Atrioventricular junction
AVM	Arteriovenous malformation
BAT	Blunt abdominal trauma

BB gun	An air rifle that uses pellets or ball bearings, made of lead or steel
BMI	Body mass index
BPA	Best practice advisory
Bpm	Beats per minute
BRCA1 human gene	Breast cancer type 1, early onset (gene mutation)
BRCA2 human gene	Breast cancer type 2, susceptibility protein (human tumor suppressor gene)
BUN	Blood urea nitrogen
C-arm	C-shaped machine used to connect the x-ray source and x-ray detector
CAT	Computerized axial tomography
CBD	Central business district
CBRNE	Chemical, biological, radiological, nuclear, and explosive
CDC	Centers for Disease Control and Prevention (www.cdc.gov)
C-Diff	Clostridium difficile
CHF	Congestive heart failure
CIN	Contrast-induced nephrotoxicity
CKD	Chronic kidney disease
CLABSI	Central line-associated bloodstream infection
CMS	Centers for Medicare and Medicaid Services (www.cms.gov)
CPH	Christchurch Public Hospital
Cr	Creatinine
CRD	Chronic renal disease
CRH	Corticotropin-releasing hormone
CT	Computed tomography
CTA	Computed tomographic angiography
CTWA-Ar	Clinical Institute Withdrawal Assessment for Alcohol, Revised
CUS	Concerned, Uncomfortable, Safety
CVC	Central venous catheter

CWH	Christchurch Women's Hospital
CXR	Chest x-ray
DCIS	Ductal carcinoma in-situ (breast cancer)
DDAVP	1-deamino-8-D-arginine vasopressin
DHS	Department of Homeland Security
DICOM	Digital Imaging and Communications in Medicine
DNR	Do not resuscitate
DOH	Department of Health
DPL	Diagnostic peritoneal lavage
DSA	Digital subtraction angiography (fluoroscopy technique in IR)
DT	Delirium tremor
DVT	Deep vein thrombosis
EAP	Employee assistance program
EKG	Electrocardiogram
ECMC	Erie County Medical Center
ED ("ER")	Emergency department (emergency room)
eGFR	Estimated glomerular filtration rate
EHR	Electronic health record
EMR	Electronic medical record
ESRD	End-stage renal disease
EVD	External ventricular drain (ventriculostomy)
EVLA	Endovenous laser ablation
FAST	Focused Assessment With Sonography for Trauma
FDA	U.S. Food and Drug Administration (www.fda.gov)
FEMA	Federal Emergency Management Agency
FFP	Fresh frozen plasma
g	Gram
GBCA	Gadolinium-based contrast agent
GI	Gastrointestinal
GSV	Greater saphenous vein
GSW	Gunshot wound
GU	Genitourinary

HBV	Hepatitis B virus
HCG	Human chorionic gonadotropin
HCV	Hepatitis C virus
HHT	Hereditary hemorrhagic telangiectasia
HIMSS	Healthcare Information and Management Systems Society
HIPAA	Health Insurance Portability and Accountability Act of 1996 (www.hipaasurvivalguide.com/hipaa-regulations/hipaa-regulations.php)
HITECH	Health Information Technology for Economic and Clinical Health (www.hipaasurvivalguide.com/hitech-act-text.php)
HOB	Head of bed
HOCM	High-osmolality contrast media
HOPPS	Hospital Outpatient Perspective Payment System (www.cms.gov/Outreach-and-Education/Medicare-Learning-Network-MLN/MLNProducts/downloads/hospitaloutpaysysfctsht.pdf)
HR	Human resources
HTN	Hypertension
HVAC	Heating, ventilation, and air conditioning
IA	Intra-arterial
ICD-10-CM/PCS	International Classification of Diseases, 10th Edition, Clinical Modification/Procedure Coding System; ICD-10 diagnosis codes are used to report medical diagnoses and inpatient procedures and were created by the World Health Organization
ICM	Iodinated contrast media
ICP	Intracranial pressure
ICU	Intensive care unit
ID	Identification
IM	Intramuscular
INR	International normalized ratio
INS	Infusion Nurses Society (www.ins1.org)
IO	Intraosseous (access to the bone marrow)

IOMC	Iso-osmolar contrast medium
IR	Interventional radiology
IUD	Intrauterine device
IV	Intravenous or intravenous catheter
IVC	Inferior vena cava
KDOQI	Kidney Disease Outcome Quality Initiative (https://www.kidney.org/professionals/guidelines)
L	Liter
LMP	Last menstrual period
LMWH	Low molecular weight heparin
LNMP	Last normal menstrual period
LOC	Level of consciousness
LOMC	Low-osmolality contrast media
LSV	Lesser saphenous vein
LVAD	Left ventricular assist device
MAR	Medication administration record
MD	Medical doctor
mg	Milligram
MIPS	Merit-based incentive program
ml	Milliliter
mm	Millimeter
mmHg	Millimeter(s) of mercury
mph	Miles per hour
MRA	Magnetic resonance angiography
MRI	Magnetic resonance imaging
MU	Meaningful Use
NaCL	Sodium chloride
NASEM	National Academies of Sciences, Engineering, and Medicine
nBCA	n-butyl cyanoacrylate
NIH	National Institutes of Health (www.nih.gov)
NIMS	National Incident Management System
NINDS	National Institutes of Neurological Disorders and Stroke

NKF	National Kidney Foundation (www.kidney.org)
NPO	Nil per os (nothing by mouth)
NRC	Nuclear Regulatory Commission
NSAID	Nonsteroidal anti-inflammatory drug
OB	Obstetrics or obstetrician
OPCW	Organisation for the Prohibition of Chemical Weapons
OR	Operating room
OSA	Obstructive sleep apnea
OSHA	Occupational Safety and Health Administration (https://www.osha.gov)
OWRS	Osler Weber Rendu Syndrome
PACS	Picture archiving and communication system
PAD	Peripheral arterial disease
PAMA	Protecting Access to Medicare Act
PaO_2	Partial pressure of oxygen
PAR	Minimum level of inventory
PAVM	Pulmonary arteriovenous malformations
PCA	Patient-controlled analgesia
PET	Positron emission tomography
PICC	Peripherally inserted central catheter
PIV	Peripheral intravenous catheter
PO	Per os (by mouth)
POCT	Point-of-care testing
POSS	Pasero Opioid-Induced Sedation Scale
PPE	Personal protective equipment
PRBC	Packed red blood cell
PSA	Procedural sedation and analgesia
PSI	Pounds per square inch
PT	Prothrombin time
PTC	Percutaneous transhepatic cholangiography
PTT	Partial thromboplastin time

qSOFA	Quick Sepsis-related Organ Failure Assessment
RBC	Red blood cell
RCA	Root cause analysis
RFA	Radiofrequency ablation
RIS	Radiology information system
RN	Registered nurse
RR	Respiratory rate
RRS	Rapid response system
SAH	Subarachnoid hemorrhage
SaO_2	Oxygen saturation measurement of hemoglobin
SBAR	Situation/background/assessment/recommendation
SBP	Systolic blood pressure
SIIM	Society for Imaging Informatics in Medicine (www.siimweb.org)
SIR	Society of Interventional Radiology (www.sirweb.org)
SIRS	Systemic inflammatory response syndrome
SNMMI	Society of Nuclear Medicine and Molecular Imaging (https://www.snmmi.org)
SPECT	Single-photon emission computed tomography
SpO_2	Peripheral capillary oxygen saturation
SSI	Surgical site infection
STAT	Immediate
STEM	Situation, treatment, event, meds.
STOP BANG	Snoring, tired, observed (apnea), high BP, BMI, age, neck, gender
SVC	Superior vena cava
TACE	Transcatheter arterial chemoembolization
TB	Tuberculosis
TCVC	Tunneled cuffed venous catheters
TIPSS	Transjugular intrahepatic portosystemic shunt
TJC	The Joint Commission

tPA	Tissue plasminogen activator
UFH	Unfractionated heparin
UIP	Union of International de Phlebologie
uL	Microliter
UN	United Nations
UNICEF	United Nations International Children's Emergency Fund
U.S.	United States
WHO	World Health Organization

Index

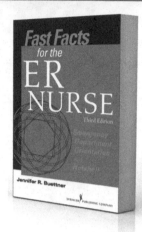
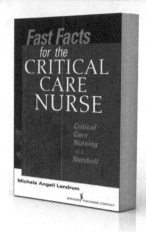
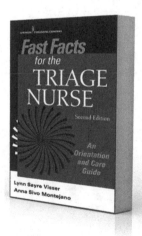
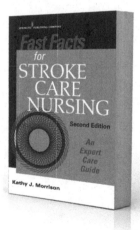

Printed in the United States
by Baker & Taylor Publisher Services